Renal Diet Cookbook for Beginners

The Proven Method That Will Help You Keep Your Chronic Kidney Disease Under Control by Reducing Your Kidney's Workload. Enjoy Many Delicious and Easy Recipes Low in Sodium, Potassium, and Phosphorus. Suitable For the Whole Family

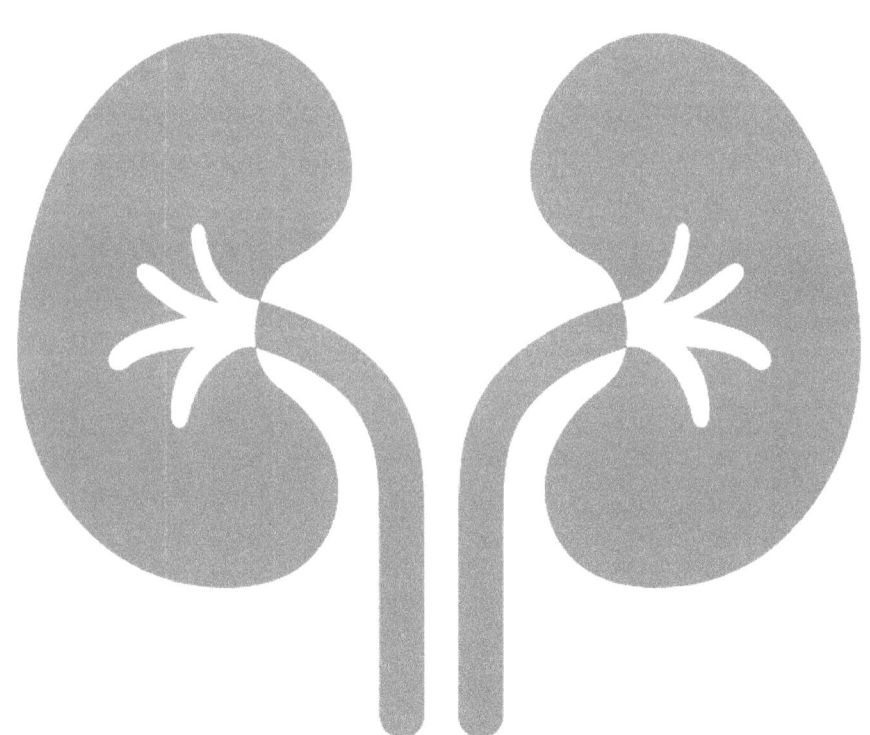

Samantha Smith

© **Copyright 2024 by Samantha Smith - All rights reserved.**

This document provides exact and reliable information regarding the topic and issues covered. The publication is sold with the idea that the publisher is not required to render accounting, officially permitted or otherwise qualified services. If advice is necessary, legal, or professional, a practiced individual in the profession should be ordered.

- From a Declaration of Principles which was accepted and approved equally by a Committee of the American Bar Association and a Committee of Publishers and Associations.

In no way is it legal to reproduce, duplicate, or transmit any part of this document in either electronic means or printed format. Recording this publication is strictly prohibited, and any storage of this document is not allowed unless written permission from the publisher. All rights reserved.

The information provided herein is stated to be truthful and consistent, in that any liability, in terms of inattention or otherwise, by any usage or abuse of any policies, processes, or **Directions:** contained within is the solitary and utter responsibility of the recipient reader. Under no circumstances will any legal responsibility or blame be held against the publisher for any reparation, damages, or monetary loss due to the information herein, either directly or indirectly.

Respective authors own all copyrights not held by the publisher.

The information herein is solely offered for informational purposes and is universal. The presentation of the information is without a contract or any guaranteed assurance. The trademarks used are without any consent, and the trademark publication is without permission or backing by the trademark owner. All trademarks and brands within this book are for clarifying purposes only and are owned by the owners, not affiliated with this document.

Contents

Introduction	5
Dietary Recommendations	7
1.1 Sodium	7
1.2 Potassium	8
1.3 Phosphorus	9
1.4 Proteins	10
1.5 Fluids	10
Food Items Ideal for Renal Diet	13
Renal-Friendly Breakfast Options	19
Renal-Friendly Desserts Options	27
Renal-Friendly Snacks	35
Salad Options	44
Vegetable Recipes	51
Fish And Seafood Recipes	59
Renal-Friendly Meat Options	67
28 Days Meal Plan	81
Conclusion	92
Recipes Index	93

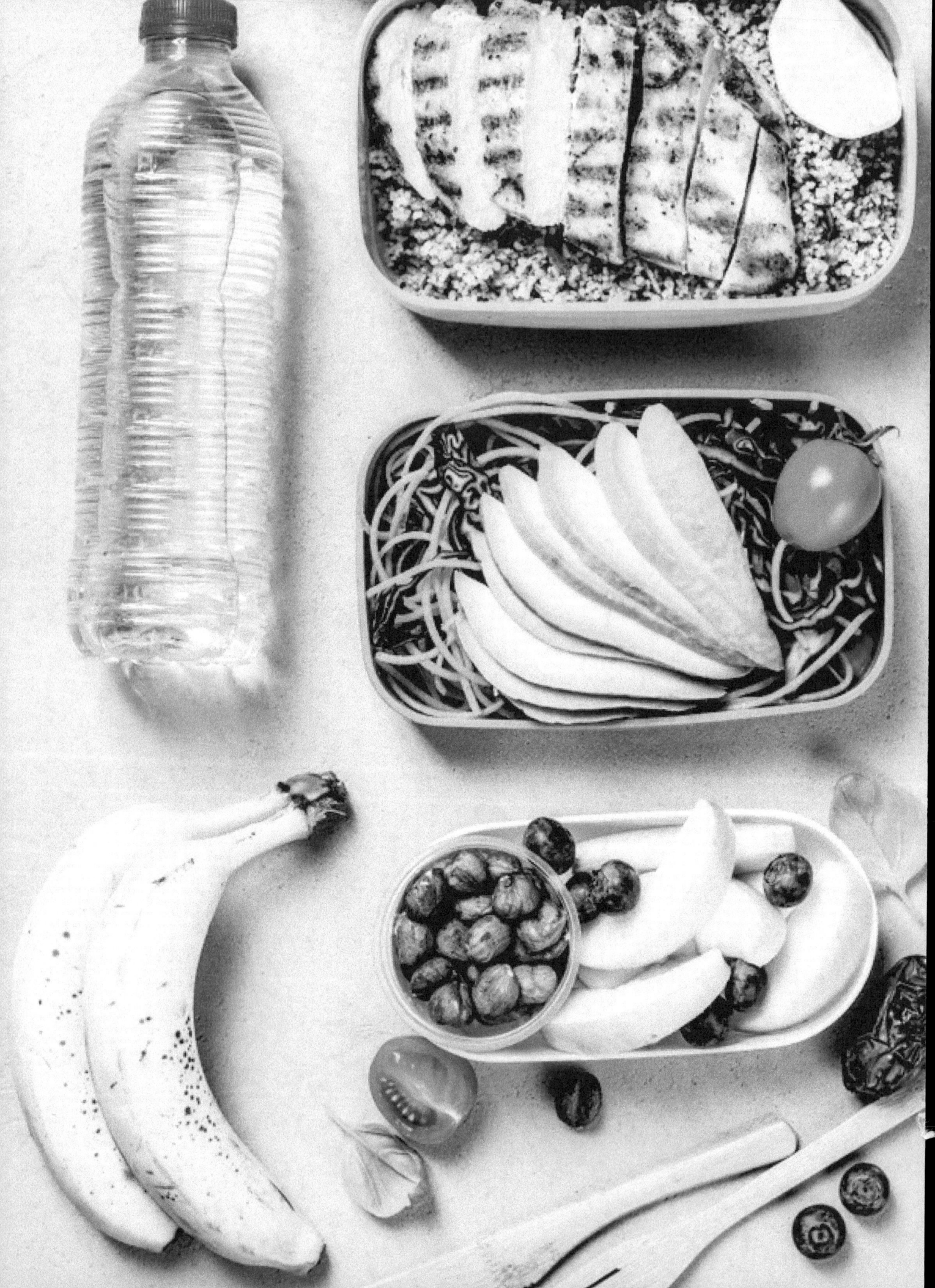

Introduction

Eating properly is essential to your therapy and may improve your mood. A new diet is an important component of your recovery. It will not only make you feel better, but it will also help you prevent problems associated with your renal illness, such as fluid retention. Overload and excessive blood potassium, bone damage, and weight loss are all symptoms of renal problems. As your kidney function is critical for eliminating food waste, it is important to note that every person will have different requirements from their diet. The kidneys excrete urea, a dietary protein, salt, potassium, and other minerals. If the kidney function is hindered, these chemicals may accumulate in the body.

A rigorous diet may help to reduce this buildup and its consequences. A low-sodium, low-phosphorus, and low-potassium diet is known as a renal diet. The necessity of consuming a protein-based diet and conserving fluids is stressed on a renal diet. Potassium and calcium limitations may be necessary for certain people. As each person is different, a dietician may work with each patient to create a renal diet tailored to their particular needs. It is important to eat well to maintain your renal health. Phosphorus, potassium, and sodium must all be limited in people with a renal illness. A renal diet is sometimes referred to as a dialysis diet or a kidney diet. Blood waste is produced as a result of food and beverage consumption. People with kidney disease must adopt a renal diet to decrease the waste in their tissues. You must keep track of everything you drink and eat if you have chronic kidney disease (CKD). This is because your kidneys aren't as effective as they should be in removing waste from your body. As a result, a kidney-friendly diet may help you stay healthy for extended periods. It is possible that adopting a renal diet may improve kidney efficiency and postpone kidney failure. The traditional renal diet is the best diet for those with kidney disease.

Dietary adjustments, including restrictions, are implemented only as needed and are tailored to the individual's age, food requirements, and development. Your calories, protein, fat, phosphorus, salt, calcium, potassium, and hydration consumption may need to be changed. Limitations are maintained as flexible as possible to help satisfy energy needs and encourage adherence. The restrictions may be raised or decreased depending on your response to the changes. In the case of a child's nutritional status, age, development, anthropometrics, eating habits, residual renal activity, biochemistry, renal replacement therapy, medicines, and psychological state, treatment via diet requires regular monitoring and adjustments. Your health is influenced by what you eat and drink. Eating a balanced, low-fat, low-salt diet will assist you in maintaining a healthy weight and controlling your blood pressure. If you have diabetes, carefully selecting what you drink and eat may help you manage your blood pressure. Controlling blood sugar and blood pressure may help prevent kidney disease from progressing. This book contains a wealth of information on a kidney-friendly renal diet and delicious kidney-friendly recipes.

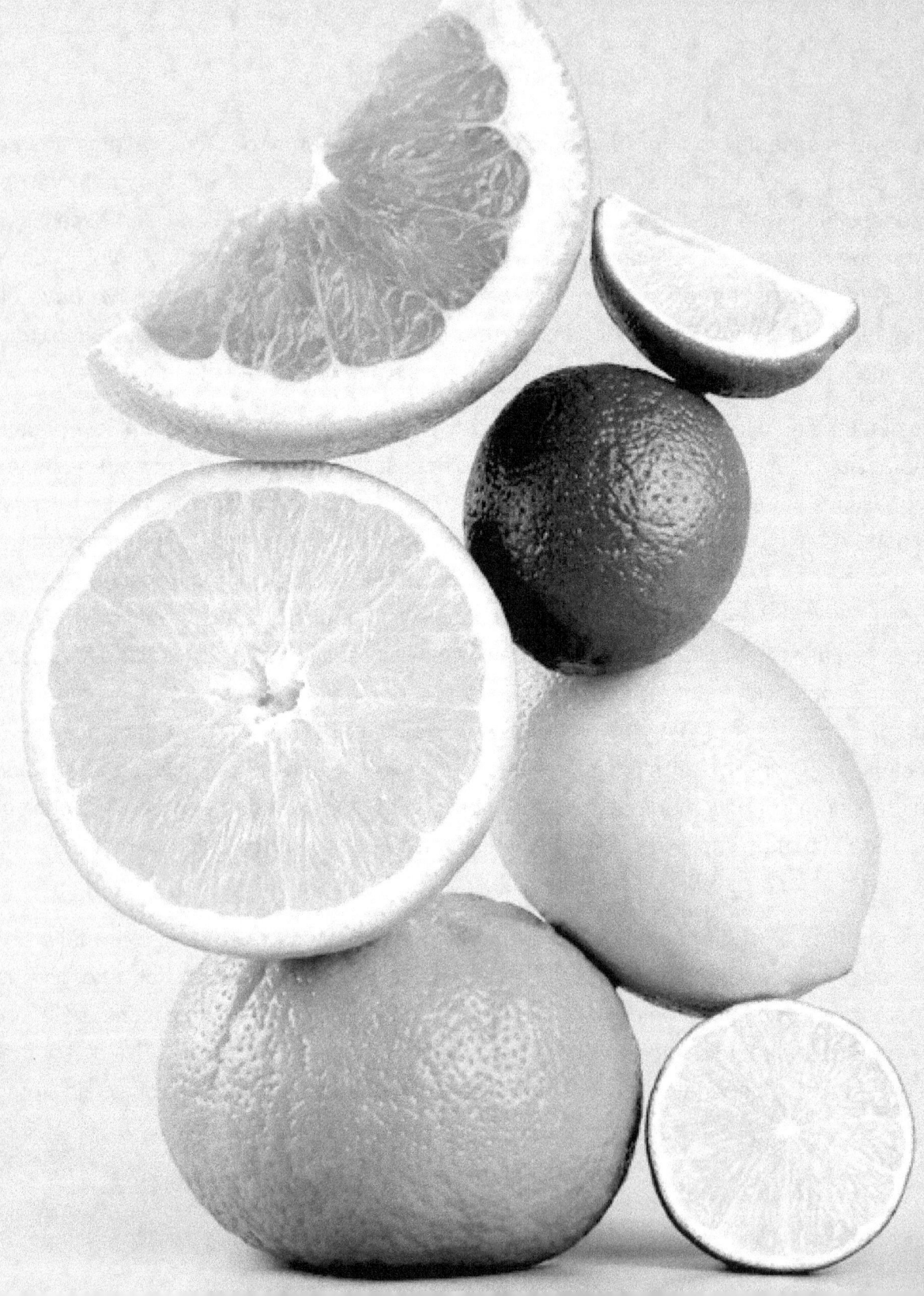

Chapter no. 1

Dietary Recommendations

A kidney-friendly diet is a way of eating that prevents additional kidney damage. It may enhance kidney function and delay the development of complete kidney failure. As certain minerals and fluids, such as electrolytes, do not accumulate in the body, you must avoid certain foods and drinks while ensuring that you consume adequate proteins, vitamins, calories, and minerals. This diet aims to maintain your electrolyte, mineral, and fluid levels while you're on dialysis for CKD. Dialysis patients must follow this diet to avoid waste accumulation in the body. A renal diet is a low-sodium, low-phosphorus, and low-protein diet. This diet stresses the necessity of eating high-quality proteins and, in most cases, reducing fluid intake. Some individuals may additionally need potassium and calcium restrictions. As every person's body is different, each patient must engage with a renal nutritionist to develop a diet that's customised to their specific requirements.

The following are some substances to keep an eye on to support a renal diet:

1.1 Sodium

Sodium is an element that is found in almost all natural foods. The terms "salt" and "sodium" are often used interchangeably, but salt is a sodium-chloride compound. Salt or sodium in various forms may be present in our foods. Due to additional salt, processed foods typically have greater sodium levels. One of the body's three basic electrolytes is sodium (potassium and chloride are the other two). Electrolytes regulate the flow of fluids into or out of the tissues and cells of your body.

Sodium is involved in the following processes within the body:

1. Heart rate and blood volume control.
2. Nerve functions and muscle contractions are both regulated.
3. Keeping the blood's acid-base balance in check.
4. Keeping a balance between how much liquid the body retains and how much it excretes.

Why should renal patients keep a close eye on their salt intake?

For individuals with renal illness, too much salt may be hazardous because their kidneys cannot properly remove the additional sodium and fluid from the body. The accumulation of salt and fluid in the tissues and circulation may lead to:

1. Increased thirst.
2. Inflammation in the legs, hands, and face is known as oedema.
3. Blood pressure that is too high.
4. Excess fluid in the circulation may cause your heart to overwork, causing it to become enlarged and feeble.
5. Shortness of breath: fluid may accumulate in the lungs, making breathing harder.

How can patients keep track of their salt consumption?

Always read food labels. The amount of sodium in a product is always stated. Keep an eye on the serving portions. Use fresh meats instead of using processed meats. Fresh fruits and vegetables, as well as no-salt-added frozen foods, are good choices. Avoid processed foods as much as possible. Compare brands and choose the lowest sodium options. Use spices that don't include "salt" in their name (e.g., choose garlic powder instead of garlic salt). When cooking at home, leave out the salt. Limit salt intake to 400 milligrams each meal and 150 milligrams every snack.

1.2 Potassium

Potassium is a mineral that may be found in a variety of foods as well as in the human body. Potassium levels in adults typically range from 3.5 to 5.0 mill moles per litre.

The function of potassium: potassium helps maintain your heartbeat and keeps the muscles in good functioning order. Potassium is also required to maintain your bloodstream's fluid and electrolyte balance. The kidneys aid in maintaining a healthy potassium balance in your body by excreting excess potassium into the urine.

Why is it important for renal patients to keep track of their potassium intake?

When the kidneys are damaged, your body's potassium levels rise because the kidneys cannot eliminate extra potassium. Hyperkalaemia is a condition in which there is too much potassium in the blood, which may lead to:

1. Muscle deterioration
2. An erratic heartbeat
3. Slow heartbeat
4. Attacks on the heart
5. Death

How can patients keep track of their potassium consumption?

When the kidneys no longer control potassium, the quantity of potassium that enters your body must be monitored. Potassium can be monitored in many ways, some of which consist of the following:

1. Make an eating plan with the help of a renal dietitian.
2. Potassium-rich foods should be avoided.
3. Limit yourself to 200gr of dairy products each day. Fresh fruits and vegetables are the best options.
4. Avoid Potassium-containing salt replacements and spices.
5. Avoid potassium chloride by reading the labels on packaged goods.
6. Keep an eye on the serving size. Keeping a food diary is a good idea.

1.3 Phosphorus

Phosphorus is an important mineral for bone health and growth.

The function of phosphorus: phosphorus is also important for forming structural tissue and organs and moving muscles. When phosphorus-rich food is eaten and digested, the phosphorus is absorbed by your small intestines and deposited in your bones.

Why is it important for renal patients to keep track of their Phosphorus intake?

Normal functioning kidneys may remove surplus phosphorus in your bloodstream. When kidney function is impaired, the kidneys cannot eliminate the excess phosphorus from your body. High phosphorus levels may deplete calcium in your bones, causing them to become brittle. Calcium deposits in your eyes, blood vessels, airways, and heart are also risky.

How can patients keep track of their Phosphorus consumption?

Phosphorus is present in a variety of foods. As a result, individuals with impaired kidney function should see a renal dietician to control their phosphorus levels. Here are some tips for keeping phosphorus levels in check:

1. Learn which foods have reduced phosphorus content.
2. Keep a careful eye on the serving size. For meals and snacks, consume smaller amounts of high-protein foods. Consume fresh fruit and vegetable.
3. Consult your doctor regarding the use of phosphate binders at mealtimes.
4. Avoid buying and using phosphorus-fortified packaged foods.
5. On ingredient labels, look for phosphorus or phrases that start with the letter "PHOS."
6. Keep a dietary diary.

1.4 Proteins

Proteins are huge, complex molecules that perform several important functions in the human body.

The function of Proteins: They are essential for the construction, function, and control of the body's tissues and organs, and they perform most of their activity in cells.

Why is it important for renal patients to keep track of their Protein intake?

Proteins are not an issue for kidneys that are in good shape. Proteins are normally eaten, and waste products are produced and filtered by the kidney's nephrons. The waste is then converted to urine with extra renal proteins. Damaged kidneys fail to eliminate protein waste, which builds up in the blood.

How can patients keep track of their Protein consumption?

Calculating protein intake is difficult for patients suffering from a chronic kidney illness since the quantity varies depending on the stage of the disease. Proteins are necessary for tissue development and other physiological functions; therefore, follow your nephrologist's or renal dietician's recommendations for your particular stage of illness.

1.5 Fluids

Water makes up most of the human body. The quantity of fluid in your blood varies somewhat depending on your gender, age, and hydration state. As the average proportion of water in human blood is about 60%, the actual number may range between approximately 45 and 75%.

The function of fluids: the fluid acts as a protective cushioning agent for your joints and organs. Avoid dehydration by drinking enough water. Headaches, tiredness, disorientation, and irritability are all symptoms of dehydration. Fluid aids in urine production and removes waste products from you body via the kidneys. By keeping the urinary system healthy, the fluids help you to avoid infections. It also aids in the regulation of your body temperature. Elderly individuals can get hot and ill if they do not drink enough liquids. Fluid also aids in the digestion (breakdown) of food. It keeps faeces smooth and regular, which helps you to prevent constipation. Fluid is an essential component of blood since it assists in the transport of nutrients throughout your body.

Why is it important for renal patients to keep track of their Fluid intake?

Fluid management is critical for patients in the latter stages of CKD. As dialysis patients' urine production is frequently reduced, fluid buildup in the body may unduly strain the heart and lungs.

How can patients keep track of their Fluids consumption?

The fluid allowance for each patient is determined individually, based on urine production and dialysis settings. It's critical to stick to your nephrologist's/fluid nutritionist's consumption recommendations. To keep their fluid consumption under control, patients should:

1. Drink just as much as your doctor prescribes.
2. Keep track of the number of liquids you use while cooking.

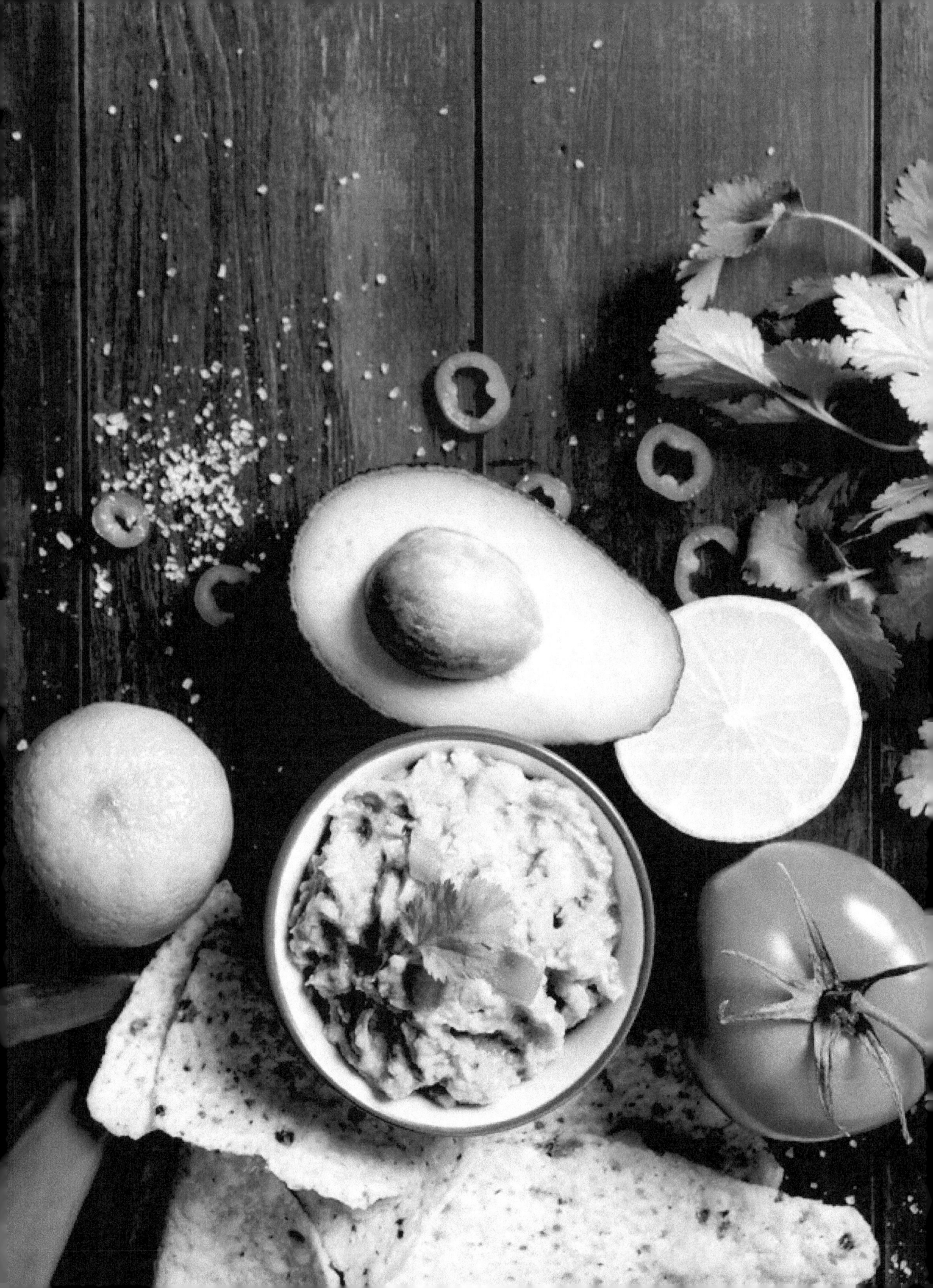

Chapter no. 2

Food Items Ideal for Renal Diet

Researchers are discovering more and more links between chronic diseases, inflammation, and "superfoods" that may decrease or protect against harmful fatty acid oxidation. Fatty acid oxidation occurs when the oxygen in your system interacts with the lipids in your blood and cells. Excessive oxidation of lipids and cholesterol generates molecules known as free radicals, which may damage your proteins, cell membranes, and DNA. Heart disease, cancer, Alzheimer's disease, Parkinson's disease, and other chronic and degenerative illnesses have been linked to oxidative damage. Conversely, antioxidant-rich foods may aid in neutralising free radicals and the body's protection. The renal diet has several antioxidant foods, making it an excellent choice for dialysis users or those with CKD. As people with kidney illnesses have more inflammation and are more likely to develop cardiovascular disease, lifestyle changes, including consuming healthy meals, engaging with a renal nutritionist, and following a renal diet of kidney-friendly foods, are critical. The following are some foods that are great for a kidney-friendly diet. Talk to your renal dietitian if you want to include these items in your healthy eating plan. These meals are suitable for everyone, including family members and friends who do not have a renal illness or are not on dialysis. Keeping your kitchen stocked with delicious, healthy, kidney-friendly meals is a big part of sticking to your renal diet.

Here are 20 of the greatest foods for renal disease sufferers:

1. **CAULIFLOWER:** this is a healthy vegetable high in vitamin C, vitamin K, and B folate, among other nutrients. It also includes inflammatory chemicals such as the phenol family and is high in fibre. In addition, potato substitution uses mashed cauliflower as a low potassium side dish.

   One cup (124 grams) of cooked cauliflower contains 19 mg sodium, 176 mg potassium, 40 mg phosphorus.

2. **BLUEBERRIES** these are high in minerals and antioxidants, making them one of the healthiest foods you can consume. These delicious berries, in particular, are full of antioxidants called

anthocyanins, which may defend against heart disease, cancer, cognitive decline, and diabetes. They're also low in salt, phosphorus, and potassium, making them a great complement to a kidney-friendly diet.

One cup (148 grams) of fresh blueberries contains 1.5 mg sodium, 114 mg potassium, 18 mg phosphorus.

3. **STRIPED BASS:** sea bass has high-quality proteins rich in omega-3 fatty acids, which are very beneficial fats. Omega-3 fatty acids are anti-inflammatory and may lower the risk of cognitive impairment, melancholy, and anxiety. Sea bass has lower phosphorus content than other seafood, even though all fish are rich in phosphorus. To control your phosphorus levels, you should eat modest amounts.

Cooked sea bass, three ounces (85 grams), contains 74 mg sodium, 279 mg potassium, 211 mg phosphorus.

4. **RED GRAPES:** these are tasty and pack a lot of nutrients into a tiny package. They're rich in vitamin C and flavonoids, antioxidants that have been proven to decrease inflammation. Red grapes are also rich in resveratrol, a flavonoid proven to improve heart health, protect against diabetes, and slow cognitive decline.

These delicious fruits are good for your kidneys since a half cup (75 grams) of them contains 1.5 mg sodium, 144 mg potassium, 15 mg phosphorus.

5. **EGG WHITES:** although egg yolks are nutritious, they are rich in phosphorus, making egg whites a preferable option for people on a renal diet. Egg whites are a good source of protein that is easy on the kidneys. They're also a great option for dialysis patients who require a lot of protein but have to watch their phosphorus intake.

Two big egg whites (66 grams) contain 110 mg sodium, 108 mg potassium, 10 mg phosphorus.

6. **GARLIC:** the quantity of sodium in a person's diet, including additional salt, should be limited if they have renal issues. Garlic is a tasty salt substitute that adds flavour to meals and offers nutritional advantages. It includes sulphur compounds with anti-inflammatory effects and is a rich source of manganese, vitamin C, and vitamin B6.

Three garlic cloves (9 grams) contain 1.5 mg sodium, 36 mg potassium, 14 mg phosphorus.

7. **BUCKWHEAT:** although many whole grains are rich in phosphorus, buckwheat is an exception. Buckwheat is a nutrient-dense grain rich in B vitamins, magnesium, iron, and fibre. Buckwheat is also gluten free, making it an excellent option for coeliac disease or gluten sensitivity sufferers.

A half cup (84 grams) of cooked buckwheat contains 3.5 mg sodium, 74 mg potassium, 59 mg phosphorus.

8. **EXTRA VIRGIN OLIVE OIL:** this is a good source of fat and is low in phosphorus, so it's a good choice for those with renal problems. People with a severe renal illness often struggle to maintain weight, making nutritious, high calorie ingredients like olive oil essential. The bulk of the fats in olive oil is oleic acid, a monounsaturated fat with anti-inflammatory effects. Furthermore, since monounsaturated fats are stable at high temperatures, olive oil is a healthy cooking option

One tablespoon (13.5 grams) of olive oil contains 0.3 mg sodium, 0.1 mg potassium, 0 mg phosphorus.

9. **CABBAGE:** this is a member of the cruciferous vegetable family, which means it's high in vitamins, minerals, and plant compounds. It's high in vitamin K, vitamin C, and a variety of B vitamins. It also contains insoluble fibre, which maintains your digestive system healthy by encouraging regular bowel movements and providing weight to your stool.

One cup (70 grams) of shredded cabbage contains 13 mg sodium, 119 mg potassium, 18 mg phosphorus.

10. **Skinless chicken:** Although some individuals with renal problems need to restrict their protein consumption, supplying the body with a sufficient quantity of high-quality protein is essential for good health. Phosphorus, potassium, and sodium are lower in skinless chicken breasts than in skin-on chicken. Choose fresh chicken instead of pre-made, roasted chicken when shopping since it includes a lot of salt and phosphorus.

Three ounces (84 grams) of skinless chicken breast contains 63 mg sodium, 216 mg potassium, 192 mg phosphorus.

11. **SWEET PEPPERS:** these include a lot of minerals, but they have less potassium than other vegetables. These vibrantly coloured peppers are high in vitamin C, a strong antioxidant. One small red sweet pepper (74 grams) provides 105% of the daily vitamin C requirement. They're also high in vitamin A, an essential component for immunological function, frequently hampered by kidney illnesses.

One small red pepper (74 grams) contains 3 mg sodium, 156 mg potassium, 19 mg phosphorus.

12. **Onions:** these are a great way to flavour renal diet meals without adding salt. It may be difficult to cut down on salt, but delicious salt substitutes are essential. When onions are sautéed with garlic and olive oil, they provide flavour to meals without jeopardising kidney health. Fur-

thermore, onions are rich in vitamin C, manganese, and B and prebiotic fibres, which feed good gut flora and help keep your digestive tract healthy.

One tiny onion (70 grams) contains 3 mg sodium, 102 mg potassium, 20 mg phosphorus.

13. **Arugula:** potassium-rich greens like spinach and kale are difficult to include in a renal diet. On the other hand, rocket is a nutrient-dense green with low potassium content, making it an excellent option for kidney-friendly salads and side dishes. Rocket is high in vitamin K and the minerals manganese and calcium, which are both beneficial to bone health. This healthy green also includes nitrates, proven to help those with kidney diseases by reducing blood pressure.

A cup (20 grams) of raw rocket contains 6 mg sodium, 74 mg potassium, 10 mg phosphorus.

14. **Macadamia nuts:** nuts are rich in phosphorus and should be avoided by individuals on a renal diet. However, macadamia nuts are a wonderful choice for individuals with renal issues. They contain considerably less phosphorus than common nuts such as peanuts and almonds. They're also high in healthy fats, B vitamins, magnesium, copper, iron, and manganese, among other minerals.

One ounce (28 grams) of macadamia nuts contains 1.4 mg sodium, 103 mg potassium, 53 mg phosphorus.

15. **Radish:** these are crisp vegetables that may be consumed in a renal diet. This is because they are poor in potassium and phosphorus but rich in other essential minerals. Radishes are high in vitamin C, an antioxidant linked to a lower risk of heart disease and cataracts. In addition, their peppery flavour enhances the flavour of low-sodium meals.

A half cup (58 grams) of sliced radishes contains 23 mg sodium, 135 mg potassium, 12 mg phosphorus.

16. **Turnips:** these are renal-friendly, and they're a great replacement for potassium-rich foods like winter squash and potatoes. Fibre and vitamin C are plentiful in these root veggies. They're also a good source of manganese and vitamin B6. They may be roasted or cooked and mashed to provide a nutritious side dish for a renal diet.

A half cup (78 grams) of cooked turnips contains 12.5 mg sodium, 138 mg potassium, 20 mg phosphorus.

17. **Pineapple:** potassium is abundant in tropical fruits such as oranges, bananas, and kiwis. Pineapple, fortunately, is a delicious, low-potassium option for people with renal issues. Pineapple is also high in fibre, manganese, vitamin C, and bromelain, an anti-inflammatory enzyme.

One cup (165 grams) of pineapple chunks contains 2 milligrams of sodium, 180 mg potassium, 13 mg phosphorus.

18. **Cranberries:** these are good for the urinary system and the kidneys. It contains A-type pro-anthocyanins are phytonutrients that inhibit bacteria from adhering to the urinary system and bladder lining, therefore preventing infection. This is especially beneficial for individuals with renal illnesses since they are more susceptible to urinary infections. Cranberries may be consumed fresh, dried, cooked, or as a juice. Potassium, phosphorus, and sodium levels are all extremely low.

One cup (100 grams) of fresh cranberries contains 2 milligrams of sodium, 80 mg potassium, 11 mg phosphorus.

19. **Shiitake mushrooms:** these are a delicious item that may be considered as a plant-based meat replacement for people on a renal diet who need to keep their protein intake low. Copper, vitamin B, manganese, and selenium are all abundant in this vegetable. They also include a significant quantity of plant-based proteins and nutritional fibre. Shiitake mushrooms have less potassium than portobello mushrooms and white button mushrooms, so they're a good option for those on a diet plan.

One cup (145 grams) cooked shiitake mushroom contains 6 mg sodium, 170 mg potassium, 42 mg phosphorus.

20. Bulgur wheat: this is a whole grain wheat product that is a great kidney-friendly alternative to other high-phosphorus, high-potassium whole grains. Iron, vitamin B and magnesium are all plentiful in this healthy grain. It's also high in plant-based proteins and dietary fibre, which benefit digestive health.

A half cup (91 grams) portion of bulgur wheat contains 4.5 mg sodium, 62 mg potassium, 36 mg phosphorus.

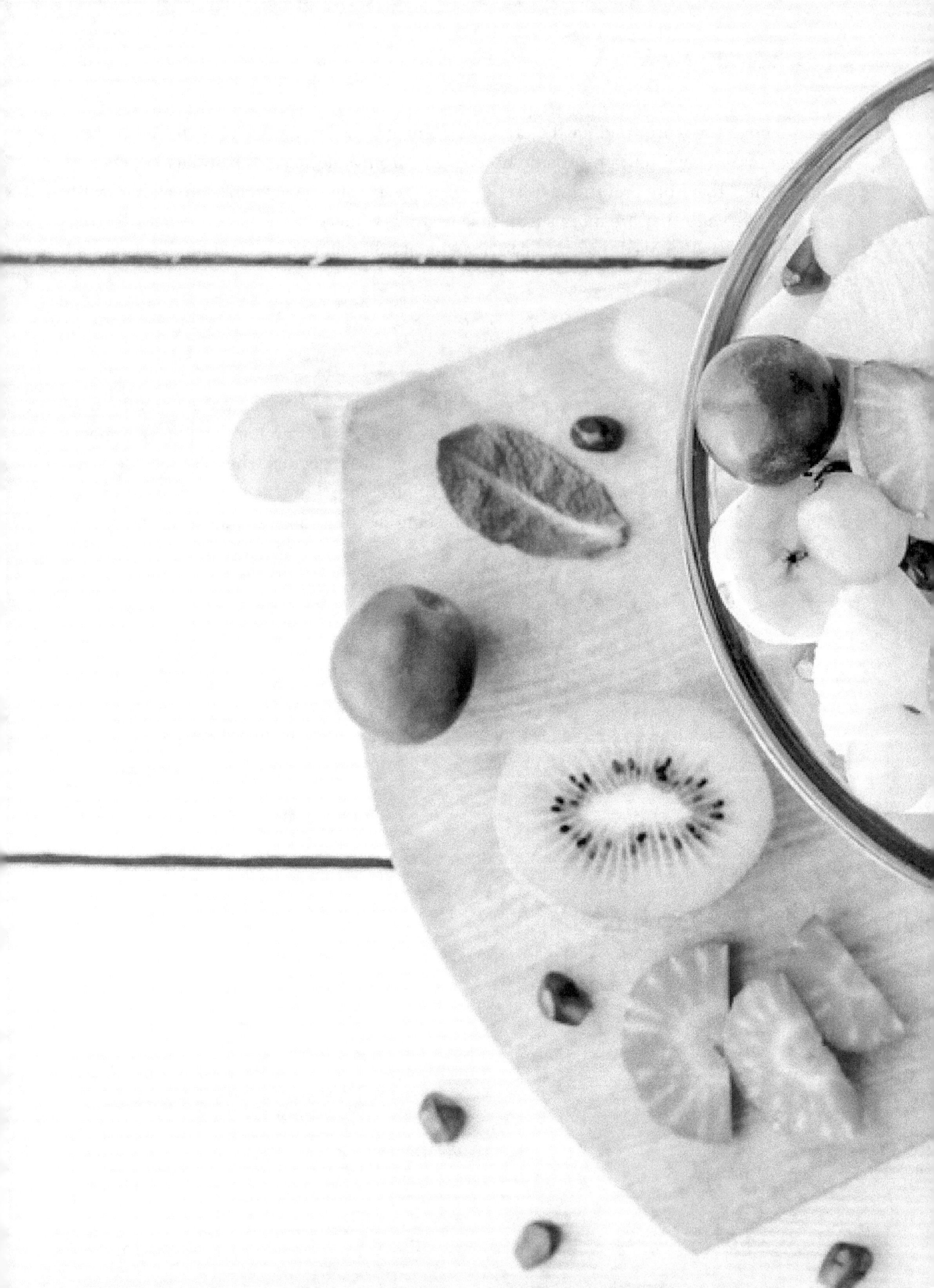

Chapter no. 3
Renal-Friendly Breakfast Options

Do you ever go without breakfast because you don't have enough time? We're here to help you out! Thanks to everything from bagels to eggs, the most important foods become the easiest meals of the day. You can quickly prepare delicious breakfasts following a renal diet plan. At least one of these easy breakfast dishes is worth a shot, so what are you waiting for? Gather your ingredients and prepare one of these quick, kidney-friendly meals to start your day.

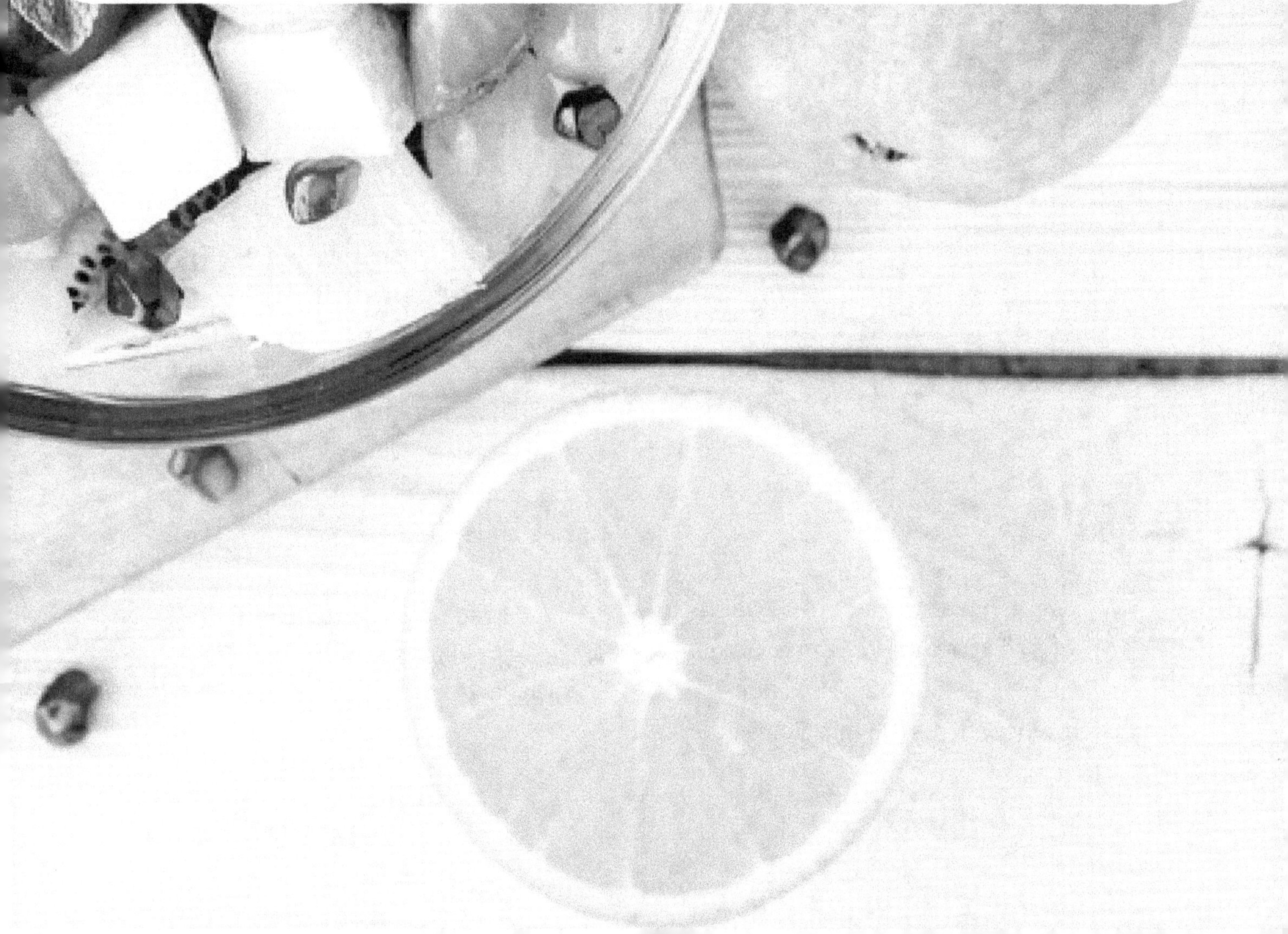

1. Fluffy Homemade Buttermilk Pancakes

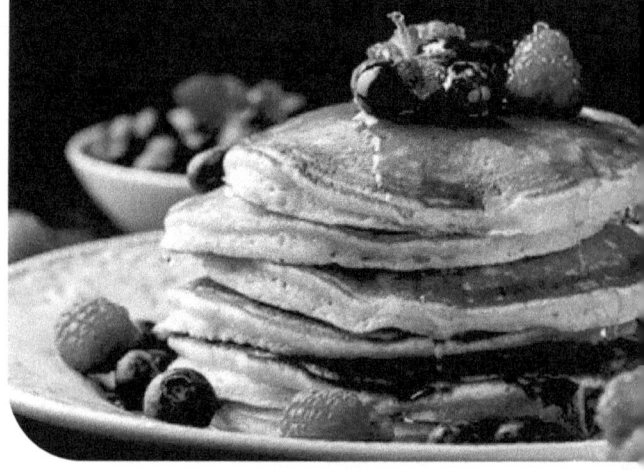

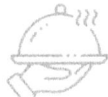 **Servings:** 9 (one serving is equal to two 4-inch pancakes)

 **Preparation Time:** 5 minutes

 **Cooking Time:** 15 minutes

Ingredients:

- 240 grams of flour
- 60 milliliters of canola oil
- 15 milliliters of canola oil
- 7 grams of baking soda
- 5 grams of cream of tartar
- 480 milliliters of low-fat buttermilk
- 2 large eggs, beaten
- 24 grams of sugar

Directions:

- Melt the butter in a pan over medium heat.
- Combine the dry ingredients in a large mixing bowl. Then in the same bowl, combine the dry ingredients with the oil, buttermilk, and egg with an electric mixer or a spoon. Combine everything until you are left with a batter.
- Use a tablespoon of canola oil to grease the pan. Using a ⅓ measuring cup, scoop the pancake batter onto the frying pan. Each pancake should have a diameter of around 4 inches. Allow around 2 inches of space between the pancakes for easy flipping. Flip your pancakes with a spatula when the bubbles on the top have almost vanished. Allow the second side to brown until the centre no longer seems wet.
- Place on a serving of platter.
- For a nutritious twist, serve with fresh berries and a side of eggs.

- *Tip:* Freeze any leftover buttermilk pancakes and reheat as needed for a quick Breakfast.

Nutrients per Serving: Calories: 175 kcal, Carbohydrate: 22 g, Protein: 5 g, Fat: 7.2 g, Sodium: 402 mg, Phosphorus: 28 mg, Potassium: 170 mg.

2. Stuffed Breakfast Biscuits

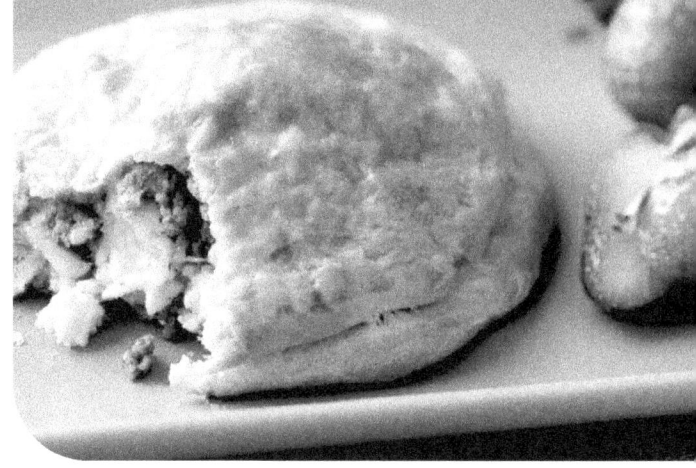

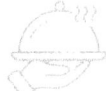 **Servings:** 12 (1 serving = 1 biscuit)

 **Preparation Time:** 10 minutes

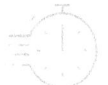 **Cooking Time:** 20 minutes

Ingredients:

- Flour: approx. 240g (2 cups)
- Lemon juice: approx. 15ml (1 tbsp.)
- Milk: approx. 180ml (¾ cup)
- Sugar (can be replaced with honey): approx. 12g (1 tbsp.)
- Baking soda: approx. 2.5g (½ tsp.)
- Unsalted butter, softened: approx. 113g (8 tbsp.)
- Eggs, beaten lightly: approx. 200g (4 eggs)
- Reduced-sodium bacon, chopped: approx. 225g (8 oz or 1¼ cups)
- Cheddar cheese, shredded: approx. 120g (1 cup)
- Scallions/spring onions, thinly chopped: approx. 15g (¼ cup)

Directions:

- Make scrambled eggs and keep it slightly underdone.
- Cook the bacon until it's crispy.
- Combine all four ingredients in a mixing bowl and put them aside.
- Combine all the dry ingredients in a large mixing dish or plate.
- Cut the unsalted butter with a fork until pea-sized or smaller.
- Make a well in the middle of the mixture and knead the milk and lemon juice in.
- Use a muffin case or gently oil and flour the bottom and sides of the muffin tins.
- Fill a 14-cup muffin pan with the batter.
- Preheat the oven to 200°C and bake for 10-12 minutes until golden brown.

- *Tip:* For a quick Breakfast, freeze the leftover biscuits.

Nutrients per Serving: Calories: 330 kcal, Carbohydrate: 19 g, Protein: 11 g, Fat: 23 g, Sodium: 329 mg, Phosphorus: 170 mg, Potassium: 168 mg.

3. Oatmeal with Honey and Fruit

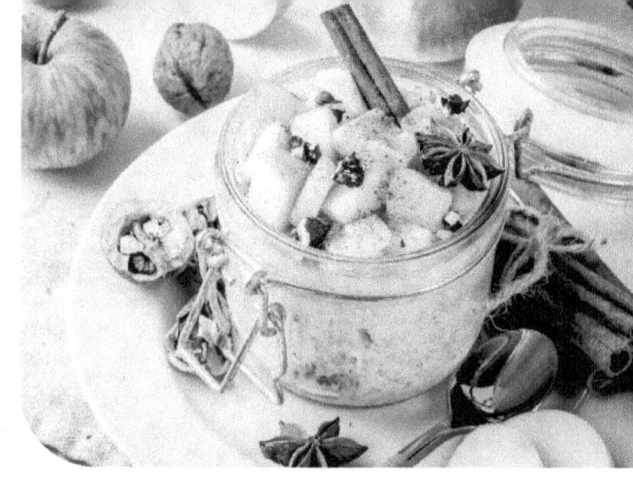

 Serving: 1

 Preparation Time: 20 minutes

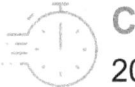 Cooking Time: 20 minutes

Ingredients:

- Oats: approx. 40g (½ cup)
- Water: approx. 240ml (1 cup)
- Honey: approx. 5g (1 tsp.)
- Low-potassium fruit (like apples or pears) cut into bite-sized pieces

Directions:

- Combine the oats and water in a pot, then heat until boiling.
- Lower the heat and let it simmer for about 10-15 minutes. Stir every now and then until the oats are soft and have absorbed the water.
- Take the pot off the heat and mix in the honey.
- Pour the oatmeal into a bowl, top with your chosen fruit that's been cut into pieces, and it's ready to serve!

Nutritional value: Calories: 200 kcal, Carbohydrate: 40 g, Protein: 6 g, Fat: 4 g, Sodium: 15 mg, Phosphorus: 130 mg, Potassium: 170 mg

4. Loaded Veggie Eggs

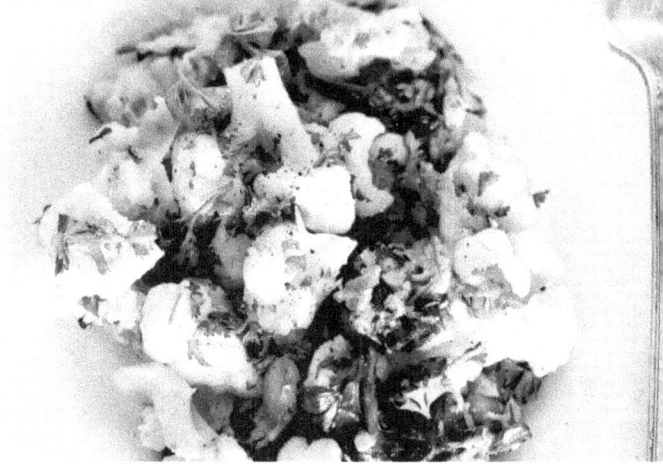

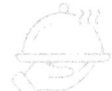 Servings: 2

 Preparation Time: 5 minutes

 Cooking Time: 12 – 15 minutes

Ingredients:

- Whole eggs, beaten: approx. 100g (2 eggs)
- Garlic clove, finely chopped: approx. 5g (1 clove)
- Cauliflower: approx. 100g (1 cup)
- Fresh spinach: approx. 90g (3 cups)
- Black pepper: approx. 0.6g (¼ tsp.)
- Sweet pepper, chopped: approx. 30g (¼ cup)
- Onion, chopped finely: approx. 30g (¼ cup)
- Oil of choice (coconut or avocado oil is good for high heat): approx. 15ml (1 tbsp.) Fresh parsley and spring onion for garnish

Directions:

- Whisk together the eggs and peppers until smooth, then put aside.
- In a large skillet, heat the oil over medium heat.
- In a pan, sauté the onions and peppers until the onions are transparent and golden.
- Add the garlic and stir briefly to mix before adding the cauliflower and spinach.
- Sauté veggies for 5 minutes, then reduce heat to medium-low.
- Add the eggs and mix them in with the veggies.
- Garnish with chopped basil or spring onions after the eggs are fully cooked. If you don't have a potassium limitation, serve with a side of vibrant, fresh tomatoes sprinkled with cracked black pepper. With these, a little Cheddar or a strong, sharp cheese would be a great addition.

Nutrients per Serving: Calories: 240 kcal, Carbohydrate: 7.8 g, Protein: 15.3 g, Fat: 16.6 g, Sodium: 150 mg, Phosphorus: 150 mg, Potassium: 750 mg.

5. Super Simple Baked Pancake

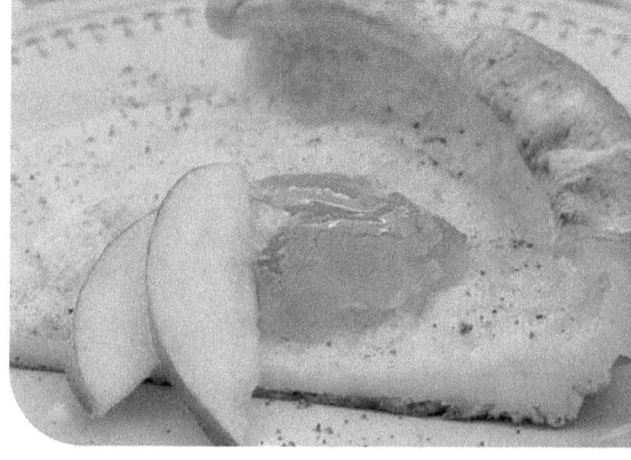

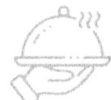 **Serving:** 1 wedge or 1/4 recipe

 **Preparation Time:** 10 minutes

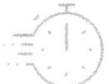 **Cooking Time:** 45 minutes

Ingredients:

- Nutmeg: approx. 1.2g (1 tsp.)
- Milk: approx. 120ml (½ cup)
- All-purpose white flour: approx. 60g (½ cup)
- Salt: approx. 1.5g (¼ tsp.)
- Egg, beaten: approx. 50g (1 egg)
- Vegetable oil: approx. 15ml (1 tbsp.)

Directions:

- Preheat the oven to 230°C.
- In a medium mixing bowl or deep dish, beat the egg and milk together using a wire whisk or an electric mixer.
- Add the flour, salt, and nutmeg, and blend until well combined (small lumps of flour left in the batter are okay).
- Pour the vegetable oil into a 9-inch oven-safe skillet or pie pan and heat for 5 minutes in a preheated oven.
- Pour the batter into the pan carefully and bake for 18 to 20 minutes, uncovered. Do not open the oven door until the pancake has swelled up and become crisp around the edges. When cooked, the middle will be nicely browned.
- Cut into four wedges and serve with pancake syrup or fruits.

- *Tip:* non-dairy alternatives, such as rice milk or a non-dairy single cream, may be used instead of milk. Potassium and phosphorus levels will be somewhat lower. Add one extra egg white for additional protein.

Nutrients per Serving: Calories: 189 kcal, Carbohydrate: 27 g, Protein: 8 g, Fat: 5 g, Sodium: 300 mg, Phosphorus: 135 mg, Potassium: 80 mg.

6. Egg and Sausage Breakfast Sandwich

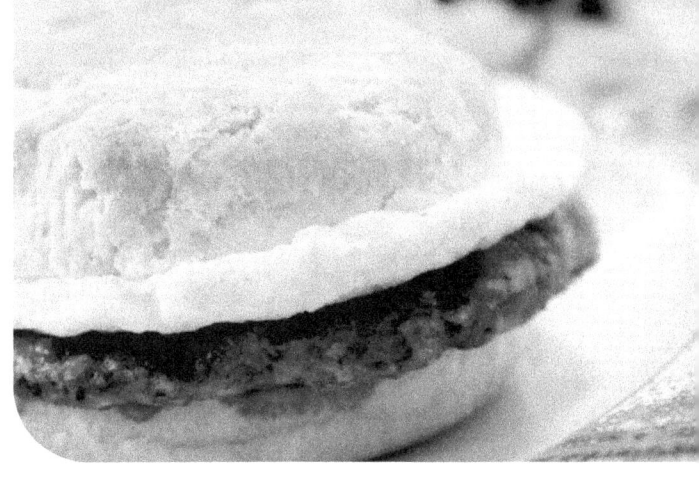

 Serving: 1

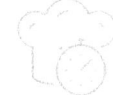 Preparation Time: 5 minutes

 Cooking Time: 5 – 10 minutes

Ingredients::

- Non-stick cooking spray
- English muffin: 1 unit
- Mature Cheddar cheese, shredded: approx. 15g (1 tbsp.)
- Liquid low-cholesterol egg replacement: approx. 60ml (¼ cup)
- Turkey sausage patty: 1 unit

Directions::

- Pour the egg product into a small pan with non-stick cooking spray and cook over moderate heat. When the egg is nearly done, flip it over with a spatula and cook for another 30 seconds.
- Toast an English muffin.
- Place the turkey sausage patty on a dish, cover with a clean paper towel, and heat for 1 minute or cook according to the package directions.
- Assemble the English muffin with the cooked egg (fold it to fit the muffin). Top with the sausage patty, mature Cheddar cheese, and the other half of the muffin.

Nutritional value: Calories: 253 kcal, Carbohydrate: 26 g, Protein: 17 g, Fat: 9 g, Sodium: 591 mg, Phosphorus: 300 mg, Potassium: 160 mg.

7. Cheese and Asparagus Crêpe Rolls with Parsley

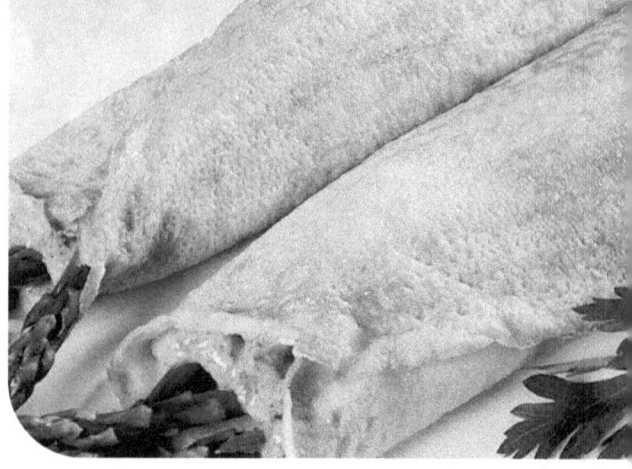

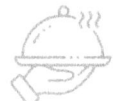 Serving: 1 crêpe

 Preparation Time: 10 minutes

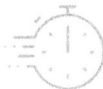 Cooking Time: 15- 20 minutes

Ingredients:

- Asparagus spears: 12 units
- Bundle of parsley
- Cream cheese: approx. 56g (2 oz)
- Egg, beaten: 1 unit
- Fresh cream: approx. 60ml (¼ cup)
- Lemon juice: approx. 5ml (1 tsp.)
- Black pepper: approx. 1g (½ tsp.)
- All-purpose flour: approx. 40g (⅓ cup)
- Fresh water: approx. 120ml (½ cup)
- Egg whites only: 2 units
- Unsalted butter (or oil): approx. 56g (4 tbsp.)

Directions:

- Steam asparagus for 6 to 8 minutes.
- For the green cream sauce, puree the cream cheese with parsley, and season with lemon juice and other seasonings. Salt and pepper can also be used according to taste. Set aside.
- To create the crêpes, mix the egg, water, flour, egg whites, and 2 tablespoons of melted butter until a smooth batter.
- In a saucepan (8- to 10-inch crêpes or sauté pan), melt ½ of a tablespoon of butter. Pour in a ⅓ of a cup of crêpe batter and flip the pan to evenly distribute the batter. Cook until the sauce is bubbling and the edges are beginning to brown. Flip it and cook for a few minutes on the opposite side. Place on a platter to cool. To create 4 crêpes, repeat with the remaining butter and batter.
- Spread the cream cheese filling on crêpes. At the end of each crêpe, equally, distribute the asparagus stalks and tightly wrap them into rolls.
- Refrigerate for one hour after wrapping in foil. Before serving, cut cooled crêpes into 3-4 pieces using a sharp knife.
- *Tip:* Fill the crêpe with shrimp instead of asparagus for a higher protein entrée. Grate the shrimp, sauté in olive oil, put it aside to cool, and then fold into crêpes.

Nutrients per Serving: Calories: 305, Fat: 24g, Carbohydrates: 16g, Proteins: 34g, Sodium: 530mg, Phosphorus: 470mg, Potassium: 870mg

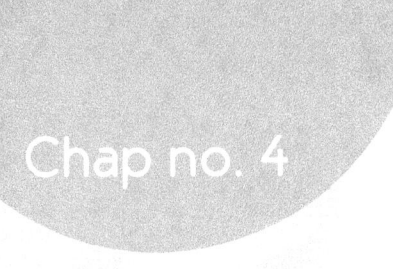

Chap no. 4

Renal-Friendly Desserts Options

Desserts help us feel full after a meal, compensate for low blood sugar and can lift us out of a low mood. Sweet foods stimulate the synthesis of the "happy" hormone in our bodies. Your behaviours play an essential part in this as well. Most people enjoy desserts, and they are also permissible on a renal diet in the same way. Here are some dessert recipes to satisfy your sweet tooth.

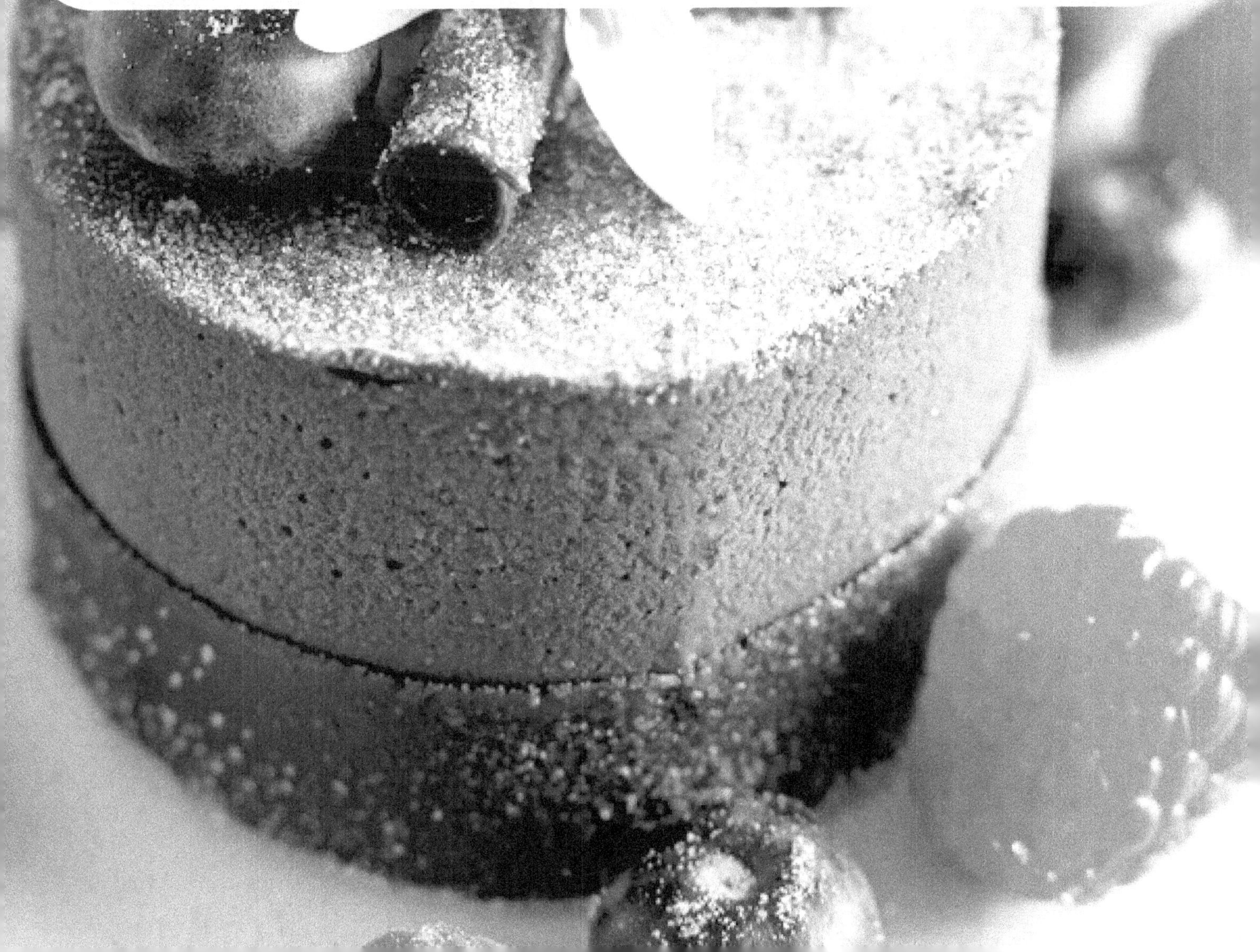

8. Blueberry Corn Cobbler

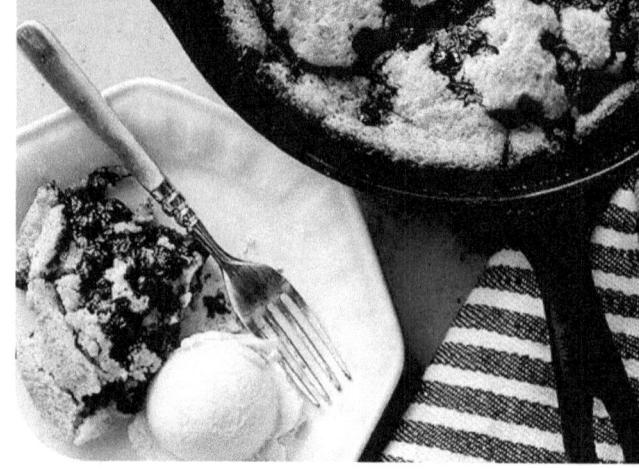

Serving: 9

Preparation Time: 10 minutes

Cooking Time: 45 minutes

Ingredients:

- Milk: approx. 79ml (⅓ cup)
- Baking soda: approx. 1.25g (¼ tsp.)
- Egg, beaten: 1 unit
- Unsalted butter: approx. 30g (2 tbsp.)
- Cream of tartar: approx. 2.5g (½ tsp.)
- White corn flour: approx. 156g (5.5 oz)
- Honey: approx. 162g (5.7 oz)
- Blueberries: approx. 907g (2 lbs)

Directions:

- Preheat the oven to 190°C.
- In a mixing bowl, whisk together the butter, milk, egg, cream of tartar, and baking soda.
- Stir in the corn flour and a ½ cup of honey until all the lumps are gone.
- In a 9-inch baking dish, spread the blueberries on the bottom.
- Drizzle the leftover honey over the berries.
- Drop the mixture over the blueberries using a tablespoon.
- Bake for 30–35 minutes, or until the top is lightly browned and the berries have popped.

Nutrients per Serving: Calories: 216 kcal, Carbohydrate: 45.5 g, Protein: 2.9 g, Fat: 2 g, Sodium: 48.3 mg, Phosphorus: 26 mg, Potassium: 155 mg

9. Proteins Booster Blueberry Muffins

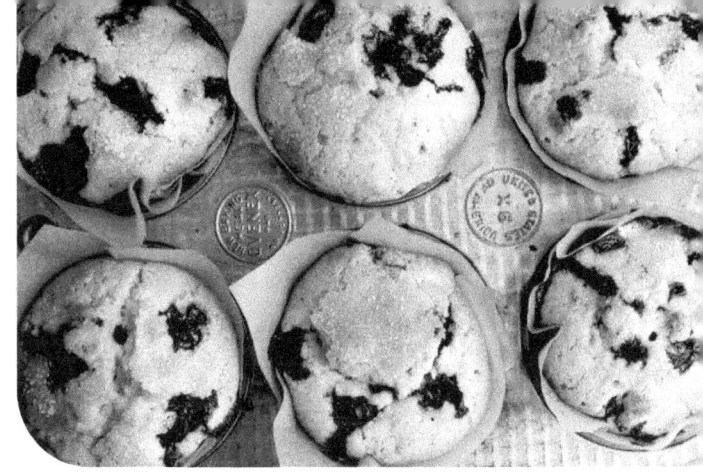

 **Servings:** 12 muffins    **Preparation Time:** 15 minutes   **Cooking Time:** 40 minutes

Ingredients:

- Butter, softened: approx. 113g (½ cup)
- Sugar: approx. 250g (1 ¼ cups)
- Vanilla extract: approx. 5ml (1 tsp.)
- Salt: approx. 2.5g (½ tsp.)
- Eggs, beaten: 2 units
- Baking powder or baking soda: approx. 10g (2 tsps.)
- Milk: approx. 120ml (½ cup)
- Blueberries, washed, drained, and picked over: approx. 340g (2 cups)
- Sugar: approx. 15g (3 tsps.)
- Flour: approx. 250g (2 cups)

Directions:

- Preheat the oven to 190°C.
- Lightly cream the butter and ¼ sugar together.
- Add the eggs in one at a time, beating thoroughly after each addition. Pour in the vanilla extract.
- Sift the flour, salt, and baking powder, then add the flour and milk to the combined mixture.
- Crush ½ of a cup of blueberries with a fork and fold into the batter. Combine the remaining whole berries in a mixing bowl.
- Fill a 12-cup standard muffin pan halfway with the batter and bake for 20 minutes. Sprinkle the 3 teaspoons of sugar on top of the muffins and bake for 30-35 minutes at 190°C.
- Remove the muffins from the pan and set them aside to cool for at least 30 min. Assuming you store the muffins uncovered, they will be overly wet the next day if they haven't all been eaten!

Nutrients per Serving: Calories: 250 kcal, Carbohydrate: 30 g, Protein: 3 g, Fat: 3 g, Sodium: 100 mg, Phosphorus: 73 mg, Potassium: 54 mg

10. Fresh Berry Fruit Salad with Yogurt Cream

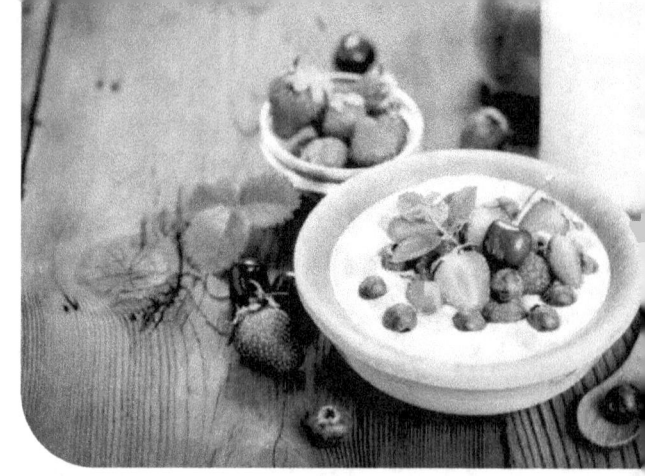

Servings: 8

Preparation Time: 5 minutes

Cooking Time: 20 minutes

Ingredients:

- Blackberries: approx. 250g (1 cup)
- Raspberries: approx. 250g (1 cup)
- Lemon juice, fresh: approx. 15ml (1 tbsp.)
- Blueberries, fresh or frozen: approx. 250g (1 cup)
- Red cherries, pitted and halved: approx. 250g (1 cup)
- Honey: approx. 30ml (2 tbsps.)
- Yogurt: approx. 500ml (2 cups)
- Honey: approx. 60ml (¼ cup)

Directions:

- Combine the berries and honey in a mixing dish.
- Combine other ingredients in a separate dish to make yoghurt cream.
- Place a dollop of yoghurt cream in the middle of each dish and top with the berries mixed with honey.

Nutrients per Serving: Calories: 117 kcal, Carbohydrate: 27 g, Protein: 3.7g, Fat: 0.4 g, Sodium: 16 mg, Phosphorus: 30 mg, Potassium 100 mg

11. Apple and Blueberry Crumble

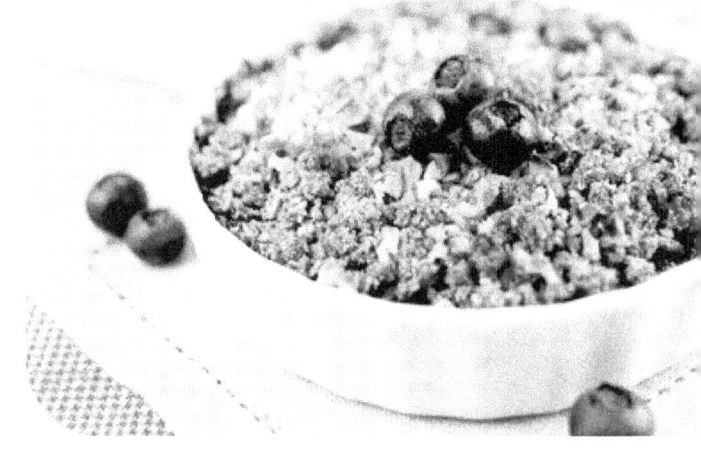

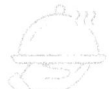 Servings: 8

 Preparation Time: 10 minutes

 Cooking Time: 55 minutes

Ingredients:

- Quick-cook rolled oats: approx. 310g (1 ¼ cups)
- Non-hydrogenated margarine, melted: approx. 90g (6 tbsps.)
- Lemon juice: approx. 15ml (1 tbsp.)
- Brown sugar: approx. 60g (¼ cup)
- Corn starch: approx. 16g (4 tsps.)
- All-purpose flour: approx. 30g (¼ cup)
- Brown sugar: approx. 125g (½ cup)
- Blueberries, fresh or frozen: approx. 560g (4 cups)
- Grated or chopped apples: approx. 500g (2 cups)
- Margarine, melted: approx. 15ml (1 tbsp.)

Directions:

- Heat the oven to 170°C with the centre rack in place.
- Combine the dry ingredients into a mixing bowl. Stir in the butter until the mixture is barely moistened. Put it aside.
- Blend the brown sugar and cornstarch in a 20 cm square baking dish. Toss in the lemon juice and fruits. Bake for 55 minutes to 1 hour, or until golden brown on top of the crumble mixture. Serve warm or cold.

Nutrients per Serving: Calories: 318 kcal, Carbohydrate: 52 g, Protein: 3.3 g, Fat: 12 g, Sodium: 148 mg, Phosphorus: 93 mg, Potassium: 180 mg

12. Almond Meringue Cookies

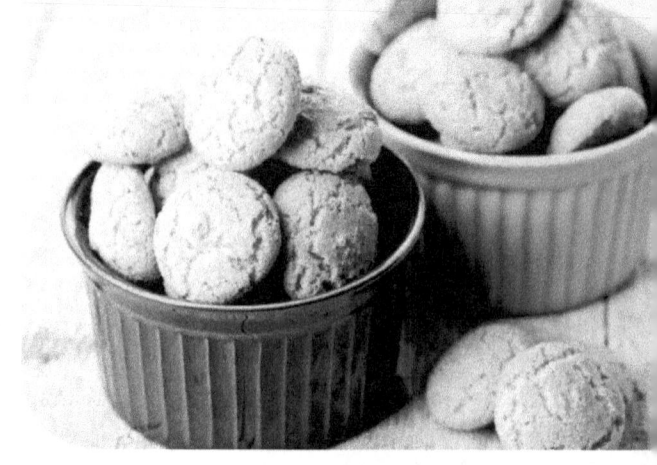

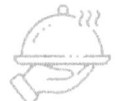 **Servings:** 24 cookies

 **Preparation Time:** 15 minutes

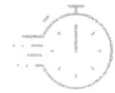 **Cooking Time:** 40 minutes

Ingredients:

- Egg whites: 2 units or approx. 60ml (4 tbsps.) pasteurized egg whites (allow to come to room temperature)
- Cream of tartar: approx. 2g (1 tsp.)
- Almond extract: approx. 2.5ml (½ tsp.)
- Vanilla extract: approx. 2.5ml (½ tsp.)
- White sugar: approx. 100g (½ cup)

Directions:

- Preheat the oven to 150°C.
- Whisk egg whites and cream of tartar together until it has quadrupled in volume. Beat in the remaining ingredients until stiff peaks form.
- Push 1 teaspoon of meringue onto a parchment-lined baking tray using the back of the other teaspoon to help you put it onto the sheet.
- Bake for about 25 minutes at 150°C, or until meringues are crisp. Keep the container sealed if stored.

Nutrients per Serving: Calories: 37.9 kcal, Carbohydrate: 9 g, Protein: 0.6 g, Sodium: 6 mg, Phosphorus: 3 mg, Potassium: 3 mg

13. Raspberry Cheesecake Mousse

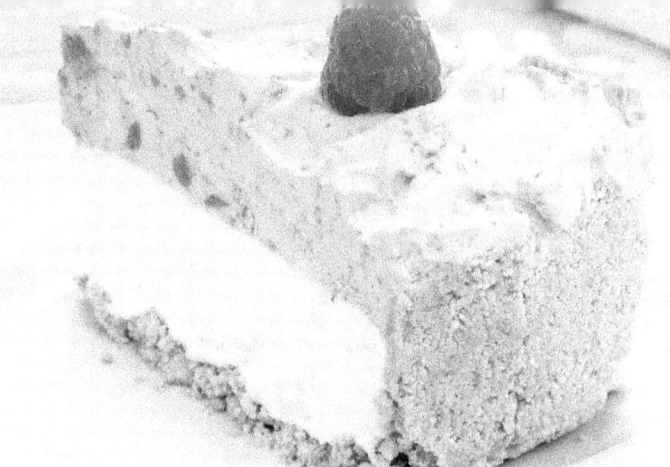

Serving: 6 **Preparation Time:** 5 minutes **Cooking Time:** 10 minutes

Ingredients:

- Light whipped topping: approx. 240ml (1 cup)
- Lemon zest, finely grated: approx. 5ml (1 tsp.)
- Vanilla extract: approx. 5ml (1 tsp.)
- Raspberries, fresh or frozen: approx. 140g (1 cup)
- Cream cheese, room temperature: approx. 510g (18 oz)
- Splenda, granulated: approx. 200g (1 cup)

Directions:

- Mix cream cheese until frothy, then add 1 cup of granulated Splenda and beat until melted. Combine the lemon juice and vanilla extract in a mixing bowl.
- Set aside a few raspberries to use as a garnish. Crush the remaining raspberries with a fork and mix granulated Splenda in the remaining 14 cups until melted.
- Fold the light whipped topping into the cream cheese mixture, then fold the crushed raspberries softly but rapidly.
- Fill 6 serving glasses halfway with the mousse and refrigerate until serving of time.
- Before serving, garnish the mousse with fresh raspberries and a sprig of fresh mint.

Nutrients per Serving: Calories: 257 kcal, Carbohydrate: 29 g, Protein: 10 g, Fat: 15g, Sodium: 54 mg, Phosphorus: 90 mg, Potassium: 128 mg

14. Cranberry Lemon Parfait

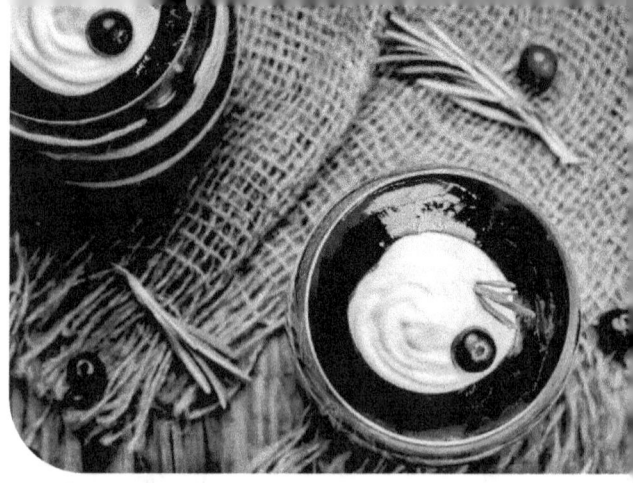

Serving: 12

Preparation Time: 5 minutes

Cooking Time: 10 minutes

Ingredients:

- Store-bought angel cake: 1 unit
- Eggs, beaten: 2 units
- Water, fresh: approx. 480ml (2 cups)
- Cranberries, fresh: approx. 225g (½ lb)
- Orange zest: approx. 5ml (1 tsp.)
- White sugar: approx. 100g (½ cup) + approx. 180g (¾ cup)
- Vanilla: approx. 5ml (1 tsp.)
- Lemon juice: approx. 80ml (⅓ cup)
- Butter or margarine: approx. 56g (4 tbsps.)

Directions:

- For the cranberry compote, combine all of the ingredients in a saucepan. Cook until the cranberries have broken down and the mixture has thickened. This dish may be served hot or chilled.
- For the lemon curd, beat together the eggs, lemon juice and its zest, and sugar over a saucepan of boiling water until the mixture thickens.
- Remove the pan from the heat and stir in the chilled butter.
- In a parfait glass, layer angel cake (store bought) with the cranberry compote and lemon curd to finish the dessert.
- Serve with fresh berries and mint as a garnish.

Nutrients per Serving: Calories: 222 kcal, Carbohydrate: 41 g, Protein: 3 g, Fat: 5.4 g, Sodium: 63 mg, Phosphorus: 17 mg, Potassium: 72 mg.

Chap no. 5

Renal-Friendly Snacks

Some individuals consume three meals each day. Some people consume six little meals each day. Others may find that one meal blends into the next. Whether you're a strict eater or a frequent "grazer", you're bound to have a snack at some point. You don't have to give up snacks no matter what stage of CKD or type of kidney illness you may have. However, you'll need to prepare ahead of time to feel good about incorporating snacks into your diet. On the renal diet, snacking is okay as long as you make good choices. Rather than consuming high-sodium foods, like a small bag of potato chips, a piece of renal-friendly fruit is a better choice. It would be best to consider how much you consume regularly. Snacking does not have to be associated with a sense of guilt. Your renal dietician will explain the best snack options available to you if your doctor advises you to boost your calorie intake. When your hunger isn't as strong as it should be, snacks may help make up for it.

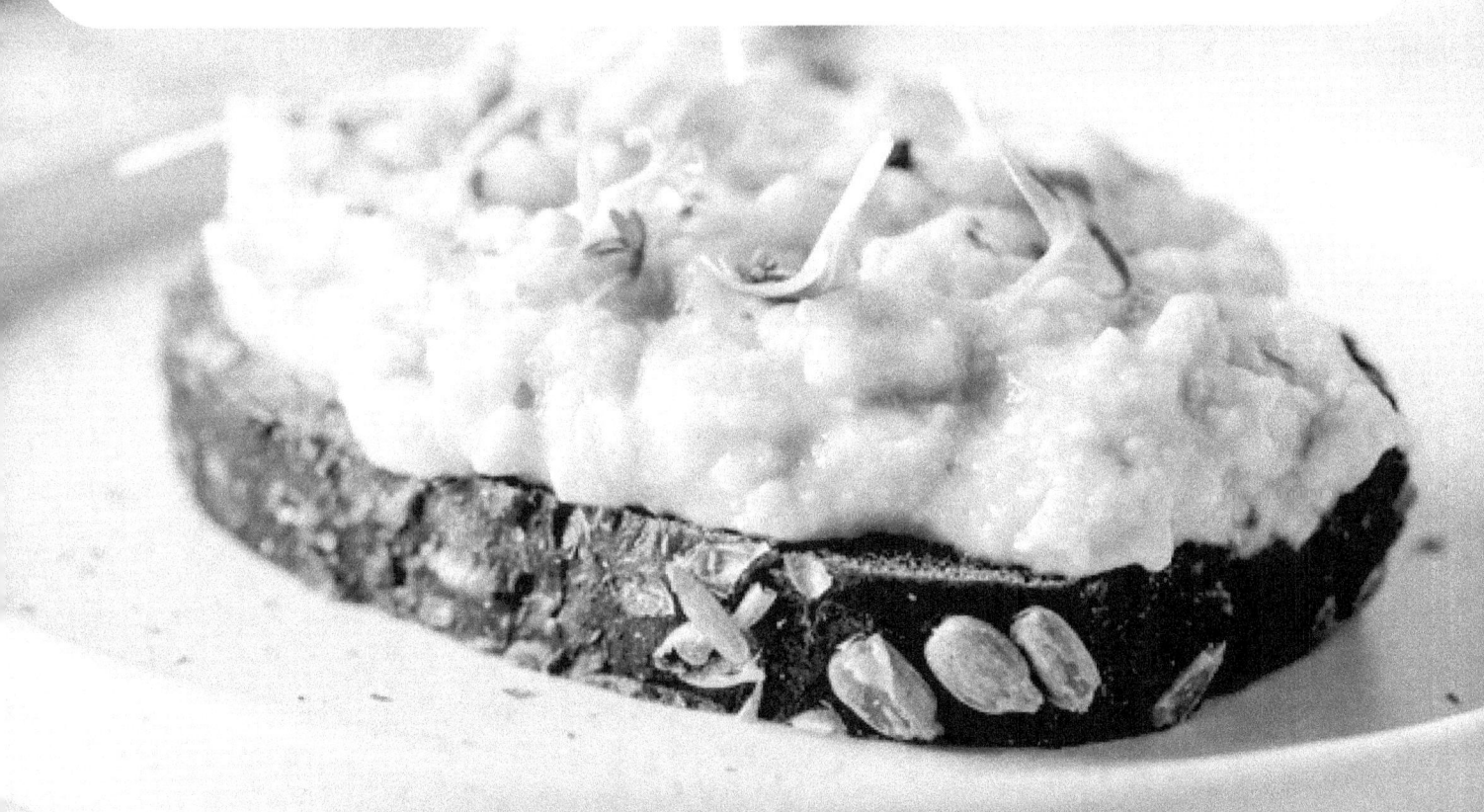

15. Cranberry Dip with Fresh Fruit

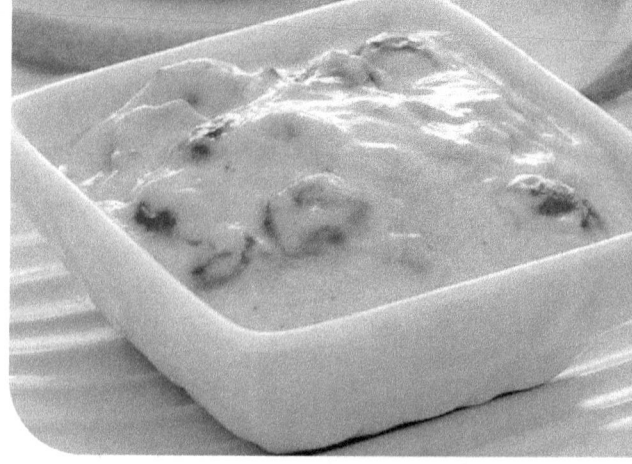

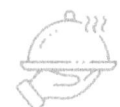 **Servings:** 24

 **Preparation Time:** 5 minutes

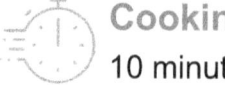 **Cooking Time:** 10 minutes

Ingredients:

- Sour cream: approx. 225g (8 oz)
- Whole berry cranberry sauce: approx. 125g (½ cup)
- Medium pears: 4 units
- Medium apples: 4 units
- Nutmeg: approx. 0.6g (¼ tsp.)
- Ground ginger: approx. 0.6g (¼ tsp.)
- Pineapple, fresh: approx. 560g (4 cups)
- Lemon juice: approx. 5ml (1 tsp.)

Directions:

- In a food processor, combine the nutmeg, sour cream, ginger, and cranberry sauce until thoroughly combined. Place in a small bowl.
- Cut pineapples into bite-size chunks. Cut each apple and pear into 12 pieces. Toss them with the lemon juice to keep apple and pear pieces from browning.
- Arrange the fruit on a plate and place a bowl for dipping in the centre. Refrigerate until ready to serve.

Nutrients per Serving: Calories: 70 kcal, Carbohydrate: 13 g, Protein: 0g, Fat: 2 g, Sodium: 8 mg, Phosphorus: 15 mg, Potassium: 80 mg.

16. Shrimp Spread with Crackers

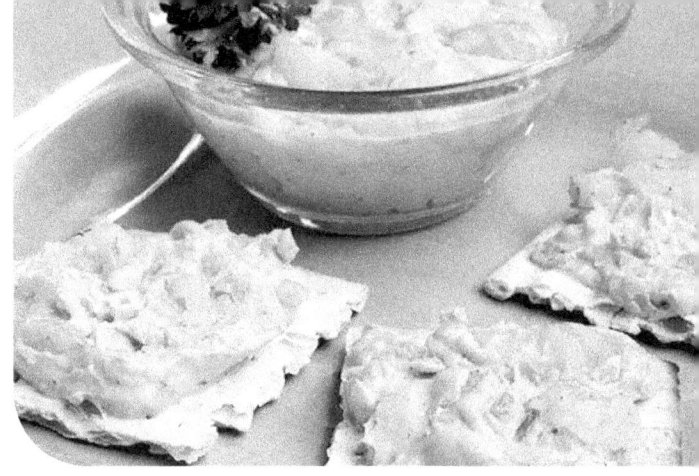

Serving: 8

Preparation Time: 5 minutes

Cooking Time: 15 minutes

Ingredients:

- Light cream cheese: approx. 60g (¼ cup)
- Parsley, finely chopped: approx. 15ml (1 tbsp.)
- Shelled shrimp, cooked: approx. 70g (2 ½ oz)
- No-salt-added ketchup: approx. 15ml (1 tbsp.)
- Worcestershire sauce: approx. 5ml (1 tsp.)
- Hot sauce: approx. 1.25ml (¼ tsp.)
- Herb seasoning blend: approx. 2.5ml (½ tsp.)
- Mini matzo crackers: 24 units

Directions:

- Allow cream cheese to soften in the refrigerator.
- In a mixing bowl, mince the shrimp and add the hot sauce, herb seasoning, cream cheese, Worcestershire sauce, and ketchup.
- Spread 1 teaspoon of the spread onto each cracker. Garnish with the finely chopped parsley.

Nutrients per Serving: Calories: 57 kcal, Carbohydrate: 7 g, Protein: 3 g, Fat: 1 g, Sodium: 69 mg, Phosphorus: 30 mg, Potassium: 28 mg

17. Soft Ginger Cookies

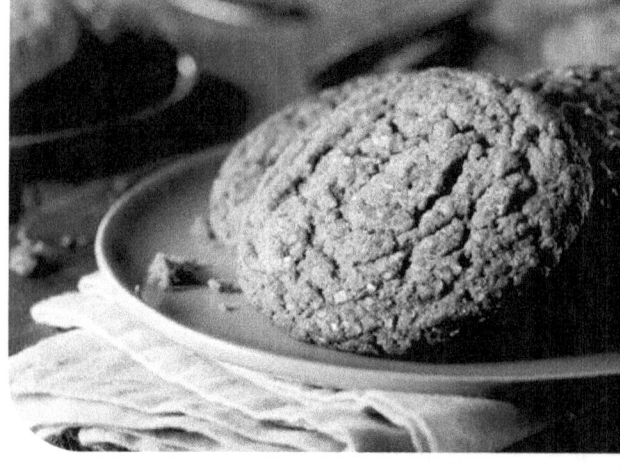

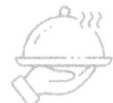 **Servings:** 24

 **Preparation Time:** 10 minutes

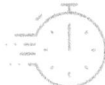 **Cooking Time:** 20 minutes

Ingredients:

- All-purpose white flour: approx. 280g (2 ¼ cups)
- Ground ginger: approx. 4g (2 tsps.)
- Unsalted butter, at room temperature: approx. 170g (¾ cup)
- Liquid low cholesterol egg substitute: approx. 60ml (¼ cup)
- Baking soda: approx. 5g (1 tsp.)
- Ground cinnamon: approx. 3.75g (¾ tsp.)
- Ground cloves: approx. 2.5g (½ tsp.)
- Sugar, granulated: approx. 225g (1 ⅛ cups)
- Molasses: approx. 60ml (¼ cup)

Directions:

- Preheat the oven to 180°C.
- Toss the ginger, cloves, flour, cinnamon, and baking soda into a medium-sized mixing bowl. Leave to one side.
- On a medium speed, whip the butter in a large mixing bowl for 30 seconds using an electric mixer. Add in 1 cup of sugar and whisk.
- Combine the liquid egg replacement and the molasses in a mixing bowl.
- Whisk the flour, salt, and baking soda in a large mixing bowl.
- 1 heaping spoonful of dough was used for each ball. The balls should be 2 ½ inches in diameter. To coat the balls, roll them in the leftover sugar and then place them on a cookie sheet that hasn't been buttered.
- Bake for 10 minutes, or until puffed and lightly golden.
- Cool for 2 minutes on the cookie sheet before moving to a wire rack to cool completely.

Nutrients per cookie: Calories: 142 kcal, Carbohydrate: 20 g, Protein: 2 g, Fat: 6 g, Sodium: 59 mg, Phosphorus: 30 mg, Potassium: 22 mg.

18. Orange and Cinnamon Biscotti

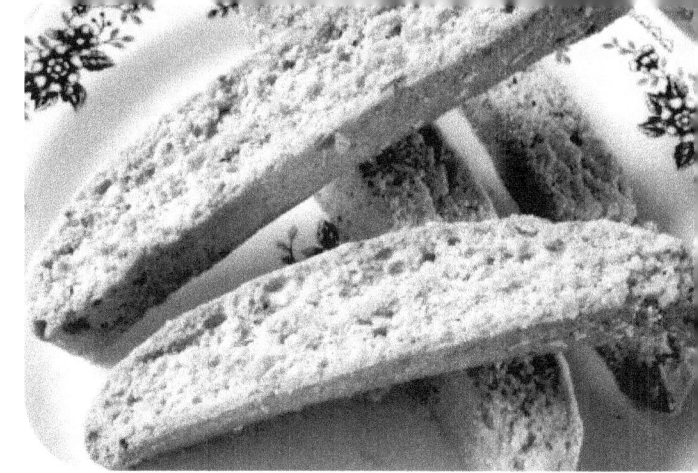

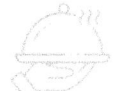 **Servings:** 2

 **Preparation Time:** 20 minutes

 Cooking Time: 1 hour 8 minutes

Ingredients:

- Unsalted butter, at room temperature: approx. 113g (½ cup)
- Orange peel, grated: approx. 4g (2 tsps.)
- Ground cinnamon: approx. 2.5g (1 tsp.)
- Vanilla extract: approx. 5ml (1 tsp.)
- All-purpose flour: approx. 250g (2 cups)
- Cream of tartar: approx. 5g (1 tsp.)
- Sugar: approx. 200g (1 cup)
- Large eggs, lightly beaten: 2 units
- Baking soda: approx. 2.5g (½ tsp.)
- Salt: approx. 1.25g (¼ tsp.)
- Non-stick cooking spray

Directions:

- Spray 2 baking trays with non-stick cooking spray.
- Beat the sugar and unsalted butter in a large bowl until well mixed.
- Add eggs in one at a time, beating well after each addition.
- Beat in the grated orange peel and vanilla.
- Mix the cream of tartar, flour, salt, cinnamon and baking soda in a medium-sized bowl.
- Add the dry ingredients to the butter mixture and mix until incorporated.
- Divide the dough in half. Place each half on a prepared sheet. With lightly floured hands, form each half into a log shape that is 3 inches long by ¾ of an inch wide. Bake until the logs are firm to the touch. This should take about 35 minutes.
- Remove the logs from the oven and allow it cool for 10 minutes.
- Transfer the logs to a work surface. Using a knife, cut ½-inch-thick slices at a diagonal angle. Arrange cut side down on baking trays.
- Bake until the bottom is golden, which should take about 12 minutes.
- Turn the biscotti over. Bake for another 12 minutes until bottoms are golden.
- Transfer to a wire rack and cool before serving.
- *Tip:* refrigerate the dough for 30 minutes to shape more easily.

Nutrients per Serving: Calories: 149, Fat: 6g, Carbohydrates: 22g, Proteins: 14g, Sodium: 220mg, Phosphorus: 150mg, Potassium 90mg.

19. Homemade Herbed Biscuits

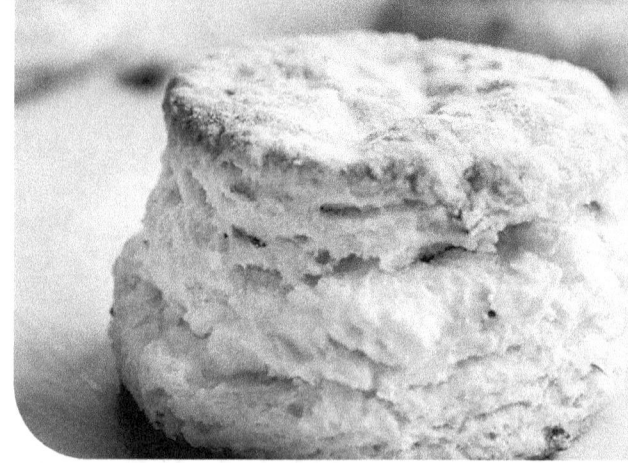

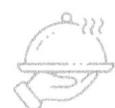 **Servings:** 12

 **Preparation Time:** 10 minutes

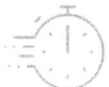 **Cooking Time:** 25 minutes

Ingredients:

- All-purpose flour: approx. 220g (1 ¾ cups)
- Cream of tartar: approx. 5g (1 tsp.)
- Chives or any other herb, fresh or dry, to taste: approx. 9g (3 tbsps.)
- Mayonnaise: approx. 60g (¼ cup)
- Baking soda: approx. 2.5g (½ tsp.)
- Skimmed milk: approx. 160ml (⅔ cup)
- Non-stick cooking spray

Directions:

- Preheat the oven to 200°C. Spray a cookie pan with cooking spray after that.
- Combine flour, cream of tartar, and baking soda in a large mixing bowl. Then, using a fork, stir in the mayonnaise until it is evenly coating the coarse cornmeal.
- Combine the milk and herbs in a separate dish and stir into the flour until everything is well mixed.
- On the cookie sheet, drop generous teaspoons of the mixture and bake for 10 minutes in the oven.
- Keep it refrigerated until you're ready to serve.

Nutrients per biscuit: Calories: 109 kcal, Carbohydrate: 15 g, Protein: 3 g, Fat: 4 g, Sodium: 88 mg, Phosphorus: 80 mg, Potassium: 55 mg

20. Chickpea and Avocado Salads

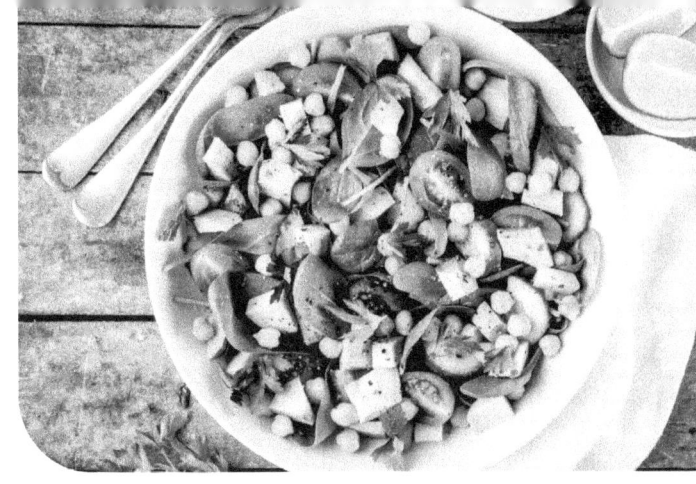

Servings: 4 | **Preparation Time:** 15 minutes | **Cooking Time:** 0 minutes

Ingredients:

- Avocados: 2 units
- Canned chickpeas: approx. 200g (7 oz)
- Cherry tomatoes: approx. 280g (10 oz)
- Rocket: approx. 60g (2 oz)
- Red onion: approx. 125g (½ unit)
- Black Greek olives: approx. 90g (15 olives)
- Lime juice (or lemon juice): approx. 15ml (1 tbsp.)
- Extra virgin olive oil: approx. 30ml (2 tbsps.)

Directions:

- Prepare the chickpeas by draining and rinsing them under running water.
- Dice the avocado, halve the cherry tomatoes, and thinly slice the red onion.
- In a large bowl, combine the chickpeas, avocado, cherry tomatoes, onion, and parsley.
- In a small bowl, mix the olive oil, lime (or lemon) juice, salt, and pepper to make the vinaigrette.
- Pour the vinaigrette over the salad and gently toss.
- Let the salad rest in the refrigerator for at least 30 minutes before serving.

Nutrients per Serving: Calories: 250 kcal, Carbohydrate: 40 g, Protein: 4 g, Fat: 20 g, Sodium: 200 mg, Phosphorus: 75 mg, Potassium: 520 mg.

21. Greek Yogurt Berry Parfait

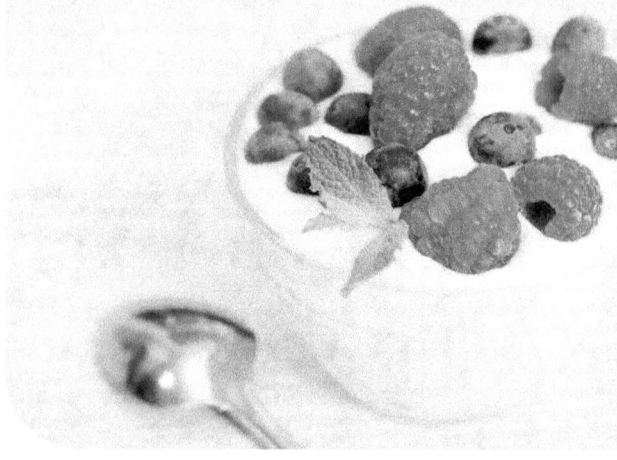

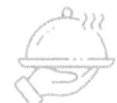 Serving: 2

 **Preparation Time:** 15 minutes

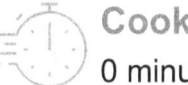 **Cooking Time:** 0 minutes

Ingredients:

- Plain Greek yogurt (low-fat or non-fat): approx. 240g (1 cup)
- Mixed berries (such as blueberries, raspberries, or strawberries): approx. 140g (1 cup)
- Walnuts or almonds, chopped: approx. 30g (2 tbsps.)
- Honey (optional, adjust to taste): approx. 5ml (1 tsp.)
- Fresh mint leaves for garnish

Directions:

- In a glass or bowl, layer the Greek yoghurt, mixed berries, and chopped nuts.
- Drizzle with a teaspoon of honey if desired.
- Garnish with fresh mint leaves.
- Serve chilled

Nutrients per Serving: Calories: 150 kcal, Carbohydrate: 15 g, Protein: 12 g, Fat: 6 g, Sodium: 50 mg, Phosphorus: 155 mg, Potassium: 200 mg.

22. Baked Sweet Potato Chips

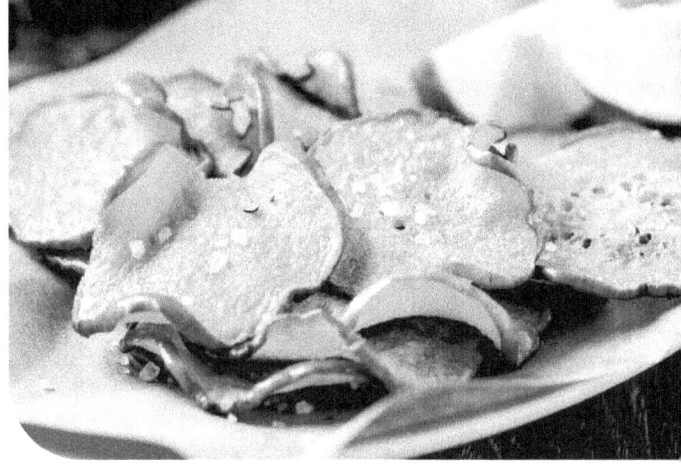

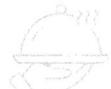 Serving: 2

 Preparation Time: 2 minutes

 Cooking Time: 5 minutes

Ingredients:

- Medium sweet potatoes, washed and thinly sliced: 2 units
- Olive oil: approx. 15ml (1 tbsp.)
- Paprika: approx. 1.5g (½ tsp.)
- Garlic powder: approx. 1.5g (½ tsp.)
- Onion powder: approx. 1.5g (½ tsp.)
- Salt to taste

Directions:

- Preheat the oven to 190°C.
- In a large bowl, toss the sweet potato slices with olive oil until evenly coated.
- Add paprika, garlic powder, onion powder, and salt to the bowl. Toss again until the sweet potato slices are evenly seasoned.
- Arrange the seasoned sweet potato slices in a single layer on a baking tray lined with parchment paper.
- Bake in the preheated oven for 20-25 minutes, flipping the slices halfway through the cooking time, until the chips are crispy and golden brown.
- Once baked, remove the sweet potato chips from the oven and let them cool for a few minutes before serving

Nutrients per Serving: Calories: 142, Fat: 4g, Sodium: 70mg, Carbohydrates: 17g, Proteins: 2g, Phosphorus: 60mg, Potassium 370mg.

Chapter no. 6

Salad Options

Salads can be eaten as a snack, a meal, or as a side dish. The following are recipes of salads for the renal diet.

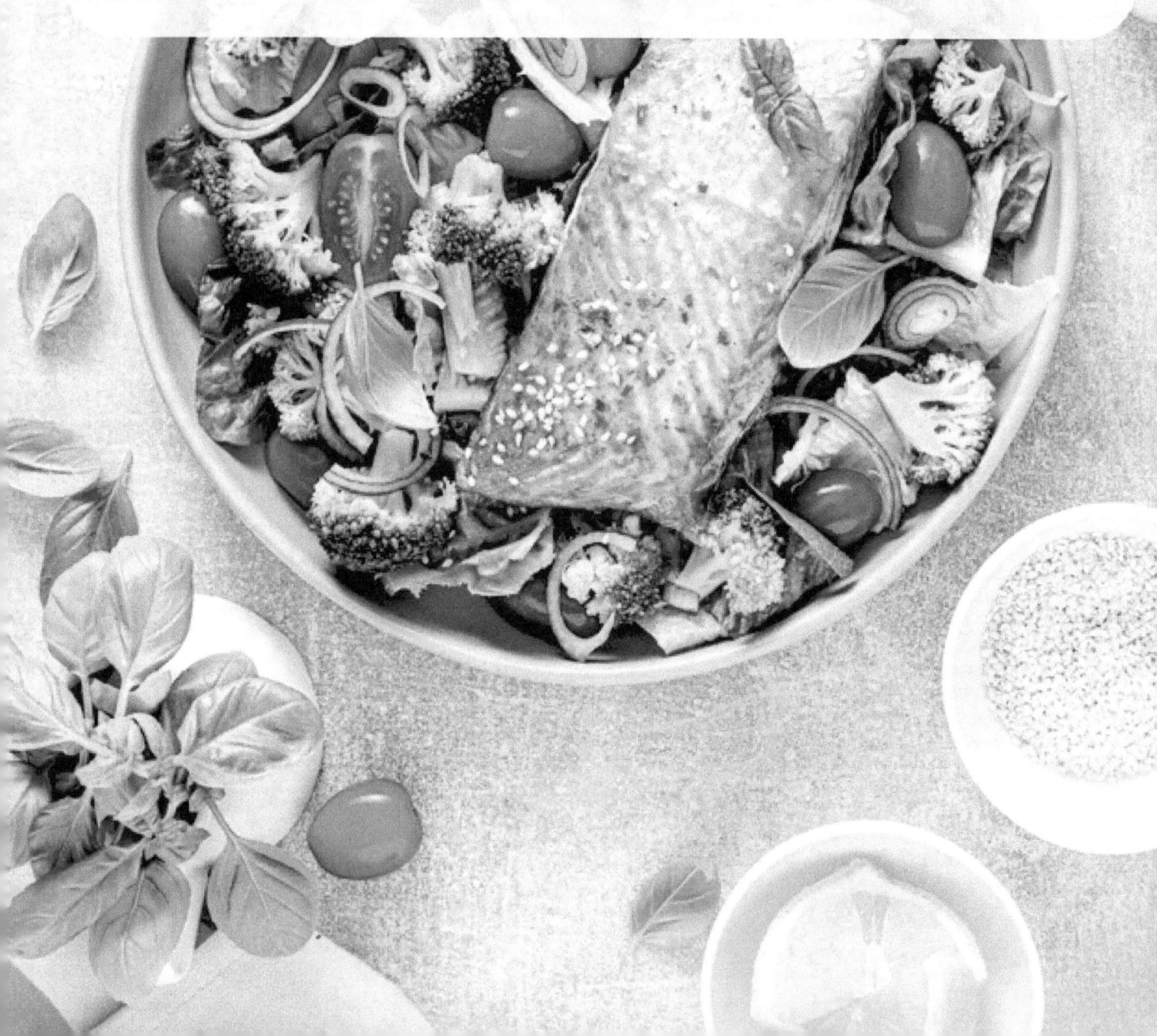

23. Salad with Lemon Dressing

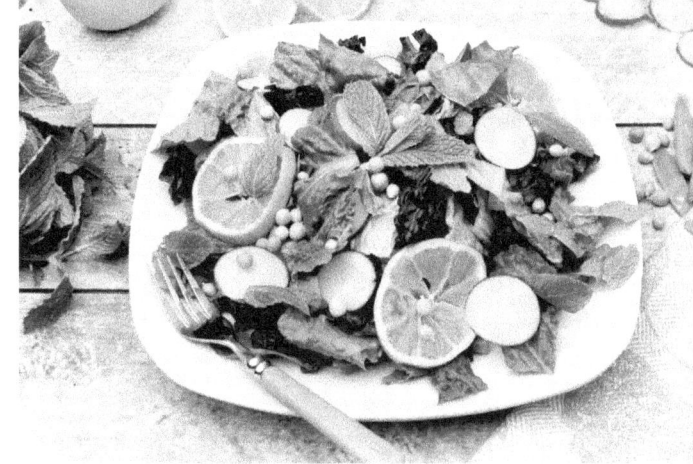

 **Servings:** 4

 **Preparation Time:** 10 minutes

 Cooking Time: 0 minutes

Ingredients:

- Double cream: approx. 60ml (¼ cup)
- Lemon juice, freshly squeezed: approx. 60ml (¼ cup)
- Brown sugar: approx. 30g (2 tbsps.)
- Fresh dill, chopped: approx. 8g (2 tbsps.)
- Spring onions, green part only, finely chopped: approx. 8g (2 tbsps.)
- Ground black pepper: approx. 0.6g (¼ tsp)
- Cucumber, thinly sliced: 1 unit
- Green cabbage, shredded: approx. 140g (2 cups)

Directions:

- Get a small bowl and combine the lemon juice, cream, sugar, dill, spring onions and pepper. Mix them well.
- Next, take a large bowl and combine the cucumber and cabbage.
- Place the salad in the refrigerator and chill for 1 hour.
- Mix well again before serving.

Nutrition Facts per Serving:
Calories: 110 kcal, **Carbohydrate:** 13 g, **Protein:** 2 g, **Fat:** 6 g, **Sodium:** 10 mg, **Phosphorus:** 10 mg, **Potassium:** 70 mg.

24. Chicken and Mandarin Salad

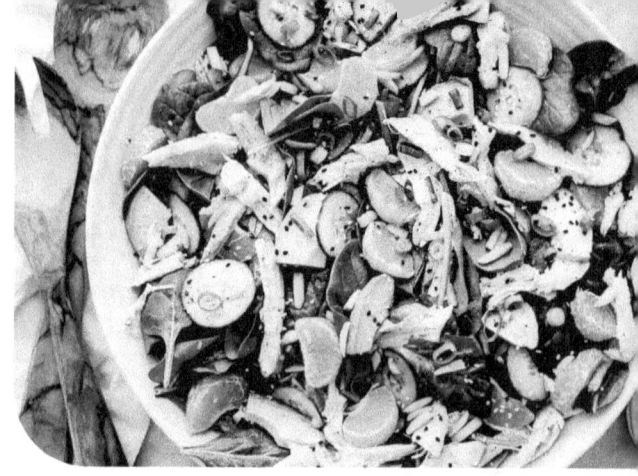

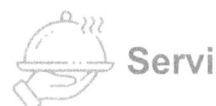 **Servings:** 3

 **Preparation Time:** 40 minutes

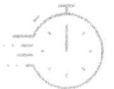 **Cooking Time:** 30 minutes

Ingredients:

- Chicken breast, halved: 2 units
- Celery: approx. 60g (½ cup)
- Green pepper: approx. 60g (½ cup)
- Onion, finely sliced: approx. 30g (¼ cup)
- Light mayonnaise: approx. 60g (¼ cup)
- Freshly ground pepper: approx. 1.25g (½ tsp)

Directions:

- Mix the chicken, celery, green pepper, and onion. Add the mayonnaise and ground pepper. Toss lightly and serve.

Nutrients per Serving: Calories: 586.53 kcal, Carbohydrate: 17.12 g Protein: 30 g, Fat: 57.9 g, Sodium: 160 mg, Phosphorus: 100 mg, Potassium: 260 mg.

25. Broccoli and Apple Salad

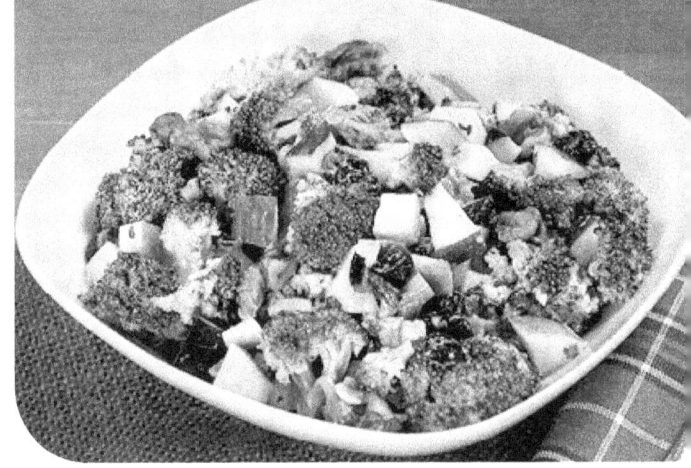

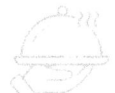 Servings: 4

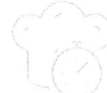 Preparation Time: 15 minutes

 Cooking Time: 15 minutes

Ingredients:

- Low-fat plain Greek yogurt: approx. 45g (3 tbsps)
- Light mayonnaise: approx. 30g (2 tbsps)
- Honey: approx. 7.5g (1 ½ tsps)
- Apple cider vinegar: approx. 7.5ml (1 ½ tsps)
- Fresh broccoli florets: approx. 85g (1 cup)
- Medium apple: approx. 60g (¼ apple)
- Red onion, diced: approx. 30g (2 tbsps)
- Fresh parsley, chopped: approx. 15g (1 tbsp)
- Dried sweetened cranberries: approx. 30g (2 tbsps)
- Walnuts: approx. 15g (1 tbsp)

Directions:

- Cut the broccoli florets into bite-sized pieces. Dice the apple into small pieces. Chop the parsley.
- Whisk the yoghurt, mayonnaise, vinegar, honey and parsley in a large bowl.
- Add the remaining ingredients into the bowl and coat it with the yoghurt mixture.
- Place in the fridge to chill and let the flavours marinate. Stir right before serving (optional).

Nutrients per Serving: Calories: 543.64 kcal, Carbohydrate: 38.8 g, Protein: 11.03 g, Fat: 42.88 g, Sodium: 40.67 mg, Phosphorus: 170 mg, Potassium: 60 mg

26. Pasta Salad

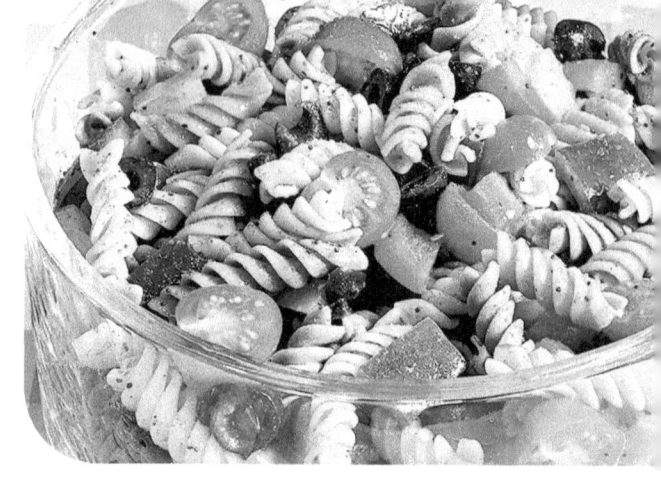

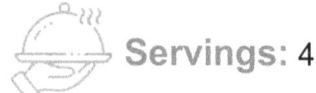 **Servings:** 4

 **Preparation Time:** 15 minutes

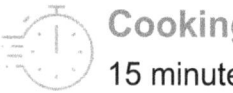 **Cooking Time:** 15 minutes

Ingredients:

- Onion, finely minced: approx. 4g (¼ tbsp)
- Carrots, shredded: approx. 30g (¼ cup)
- Broccoli florets: approx. 30g (¼ cup)
- Cucumber, diced: approx. 30g (¼ cup)
- Red sweet pepper, chopped: approx. 30g (¼ cup)
- Distilled white vinegar: approx. 30ml (2 tbsps)
- Olive oil: approx. 30ml (2 tbsps)
- Garlic powder: a pinch
- Black pepper: a pinch
- Dried oregano: approx. 0.3g (⅛ tsp)
- Celery seed: approx. 0.3g (⅛ tsp)
- Rotini pasta: approx. 57g (2 oz)
- Grated Parmesan cheese: approx. 5g (1 tbsp)
- Herb seasoning blend: approx. 0.6g (¼ tsp)
- Paprika: a pinch

Directions:

- Cut the broccoli florets into small pieces. Set aside.
- To make the dressing, combine the vinegar, oregano, oil, pepper, garlic powder, celery seed, and onion. Set aside.
- Cook the pasta until it is al dente.
- Drain the pasta, rinse, then toss with enough dressing to coat the pasta entirely.
- Add the Parmesan cheese to the pasta and refrigerate for at least 12 hours.
- Add the remaining vegetables, herb seasoning blend, and paprika, and toss 2 hours before serving. Add more dressing if needed or desired.
- Refrigerate until ready to serve.

Nutrients per Serving: Calories: 201.81 kcal, Carbohydrate: 20.68 g, Protein: 2.99 g, Fat: 14.44 g, Sodium: 93.79 mg, Phosphorus: 74 mg.

27. Roasted Red Pepper Hummus with Veggie Sticks

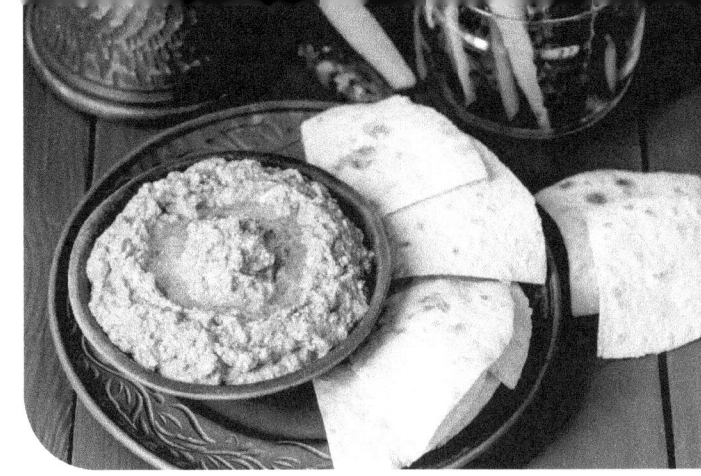

Servings: 2

Preparation Time: 15 minutes

Cooking Time: 0 minutes

Ingredients:

- Canned chickpeas, rinsed and drained: approx. 200g (1 cup)
- Large roasted red sweet pepper, store-bought or homemade: 1 unit
- Garlic cloves, minced: 2 units.
- Tahini (sesame seed paste): approx. 30g (2 tbsps)
- Juice of 1 lemon
- Extra-virgin olive oil: approx. 15ml (1 tbsp)
- Salt and pepper to taste
- Assorted veggie sticks (carrot, celery, cucumber, etc.) for dipping

Directions:

- In a food processor, combine the chickpeas, roasted red pepper, minced garlic, tahini, lemon juice, and olive oil.
- Blend until smooth, adding a splash of water if needed to achieve the desired consistency.
- Season with salt and pepper to taste.
- Serve the roasted red pepper hummus with the veggie sticks for dipping.

Nutrients per Serving: Calories: 160 kcal, Carbohydrate: 27 g, Protein: 7 g, Fat: 6g, Sodium: 200 mg, Phosphorus: 100 mg, Potassium: 250 mg.

28. Turkey Salad

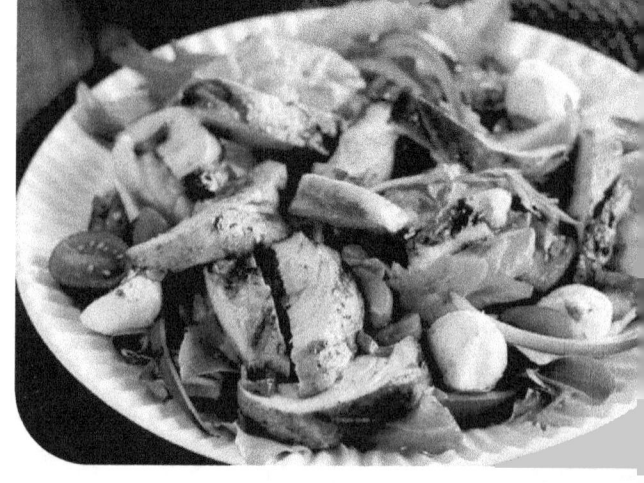

Servings: 2

Preparation Time: 15 minutes

Cooking Time: 15 minutes

Ingredients:

- Cooked, unsalted turkey breast, cubed: approx. 113g (4 oz)
- Medium red apple, diced: 1 unit
- Celery, diced: approx. 55g (⅓ cup)
- Onion, finely chopped: approx. 20g (2 tbsps + 2 tsps)
- Mayonnaise: approx. 20g (1 tbsp + 1 tsp)
- Apple juice: approx. 10ml (2 tsps)

Directions:

- Add all ingredients into a medium bowl. Stir together until well mixed.
- Chill until ready to serve.

Nutrients per Serving: Calories: 748.28 kcal, Carbohydrate: 29.26 g, Protein: 12.78 g, Fat: 65.47 g, Sodium: 120 mg, Phosphorus: 100 mg, Potassium: 189 mg..

Chapter no. 7

Vegetable Recipes

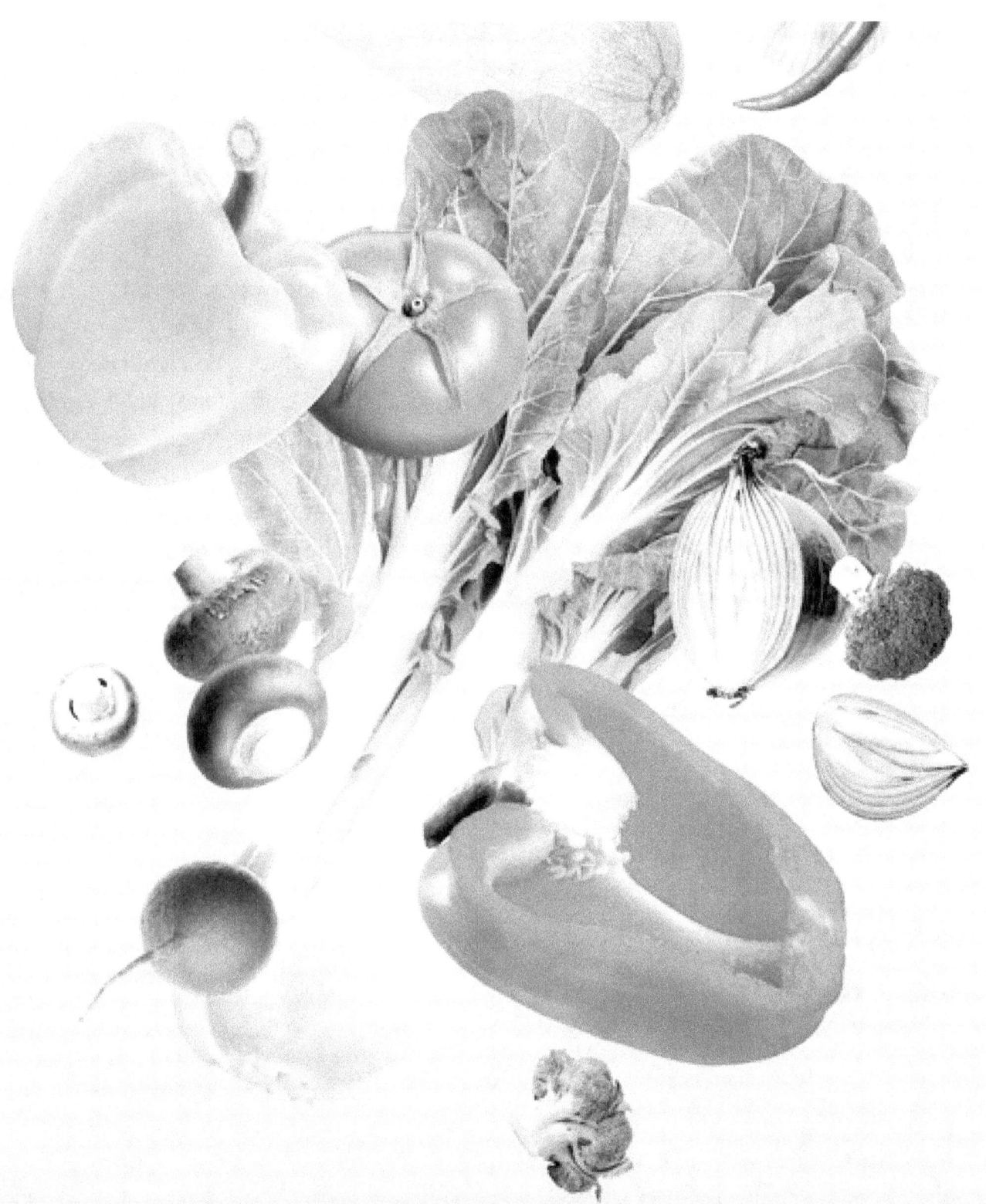

29. Glazed Snap Peas

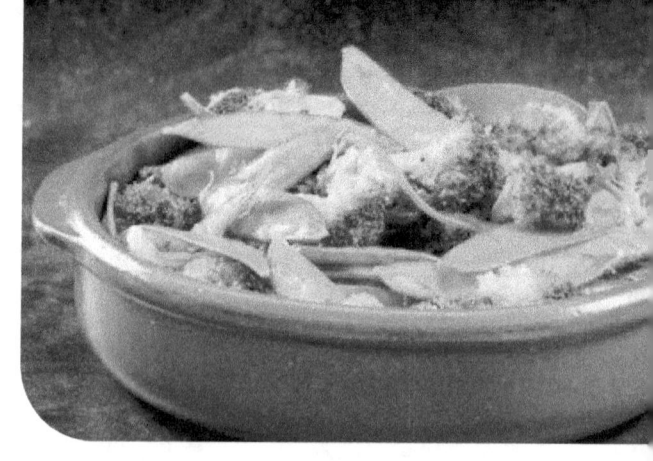

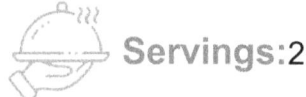 Servings: 2

 **Preparation Time:** 10 minutes

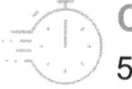 **Cooking Time:** 5 minutes

Ingredients:

- Snap peas: approx. 160g (1 cup)
- Erythritol: approx. 8g (2 tsp)
- Butter, melted: approx. 5ml (1 tsp)
- Ground nutmeg: approx. 1.5g (¾ tsp)
- Salt: approx. 1.5g (¼ tsp)
- Water: approx. 240ml (1 cup)

Directions:

- Pour the water into the pan. Add snap peas and bring them to a boil.
- Boil the snap peas for 5 minutes over a medium heat.
- Then drain the water and chill the snap peas.
- Meanwhile, whisk the ground nutmeg, melted butter, salt, and erythritol together.
- Heat the mixture in the microwave for 5 seconds.
- Pour the sweet, buttery liquid over the snap peas and shake them well.
- The side dish should only be served warm.

Nutrition Per Serving: Calories 64 kcal, Carbohydrate: 7.1 g, Protein: 2.8 g, Fat: 3.1 g, Sodium: 75 mg, Phosphorus: 110 mg, Potassium: 170 mg

30. Vegetable Masala

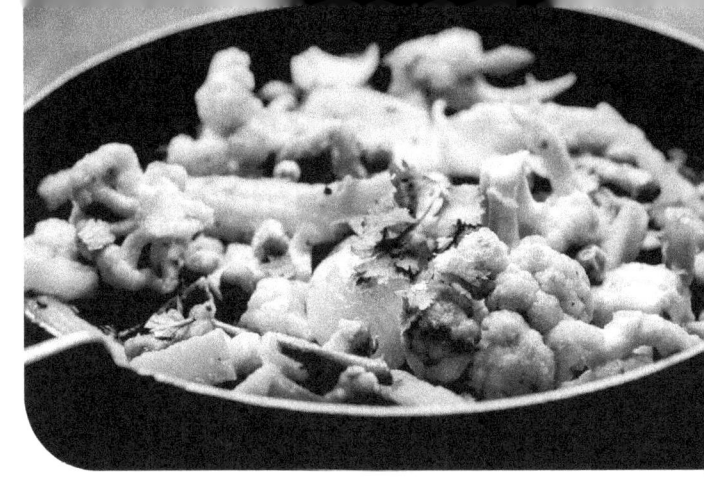

Preparation Time: 10 minutes

Cooking Time: 18 minutes

Servings: 4

Ingredients:

- Green beans, chopped: approx. 260g (2 cups)
- White mushroom, chopped: approx. 120g (1 cup)
- Garlic, minced: approx. 5g (1 tsp)
- Ginger, minced: approx. 5g (1 tsp)
- Chili flakes: approx. 2.5g (1 tsp)
- Garam masala: approx. 6g (1 tbsp)
- Olive oil: approx. 15ml (1 tbsp)
- Salt: approx. 2,5g (1/2 tsp)

Directions:

- Line the tray with baking paper and preheat the oven to 180°C.
- Place the green beans and mushrooms on the tray.
- Sprinkle the vegetables with the minced garlic, ginger, chili flakes, garam masala, olive oil, and salt.
- Mix well so the green beans and mushrooms are coated, and transfer to the oven.
- Cook vegetable masala for 18 minutes.

Nutrients per Serving: Calories 81 kcal, Carbohydrate: 11.1 g, Protein: 1.9 g, Fat: 4.2 g, Sodium: 75 mg, Phosphorus: 110 mg, Potassium: 280 mg.

31. Cilantro Chili Burgers

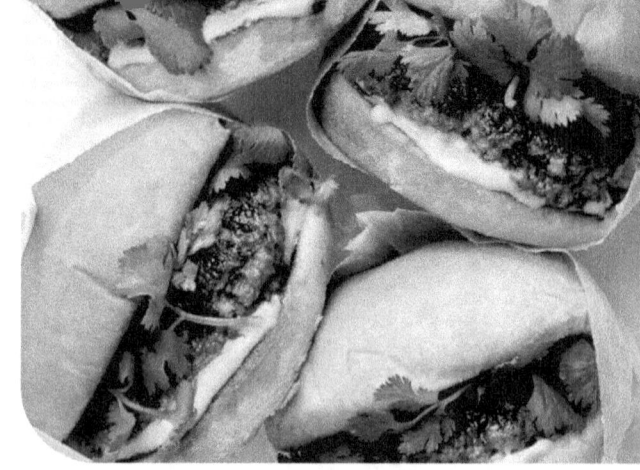

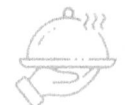 **Servings:** 3

 **Preparation Time:** 10 minutes

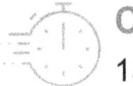 **Cooking Time:** 15 minutes

Ingredients:

- Red cabbage: approx. 90g (1 cup)
- Almond flour: approx. 27g (3 tbsps)
- Cream cheese: approx. 15g (1 tbsp)
- Spring onions, chopped: approx. 28g (1 oz)
- Salt: approx. 2.5g (½ tsp)
- Chili powder: approx. 2.5g (½ tsp)
- Fresh coriander: approx. 8g (½ cup)

Directions:

- Chop red cabbage roughly and transfer it to the blender.
- Add fresh coriander and blend the mixture until very smooth. Then, transfer it into a bowl.
- Add cream cheese, spring onions, salt, chili powder, and almond flour.
- Stir the mixture well.
- Make 3 big burgers from the cabbage mixture or 6 small burgers.
- Line the baking tray with baking paper.
- Place the burgers on the tray.
- Bake the coriander burgers for 15 minutes at 180°C.
- Flip the burgers onto another side after 8 minutes of cooking.

Nutrients per Serving: Calories: 227 kcal, Carbohydrate: 9.5 g, Proteins 9.9 g, Fat: 18.6 g, Sodium: 95 mg, Phosphorus: 116 mg, Potassium: 200 mg

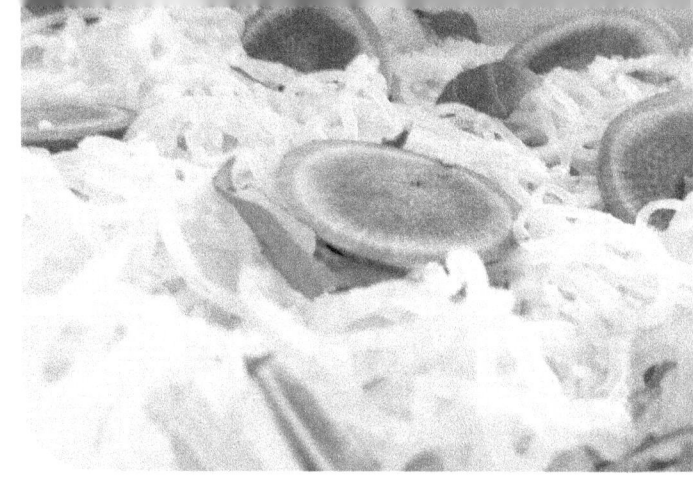

32. Jicama Noodles

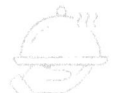 Servings: 6

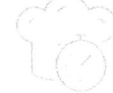 Preparation Time: 15 minutes

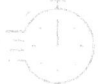 Cooking Time: 7 minutes

Ingredients:

- Jicama, peeled: approx. 454g (1 lb)
- Butter: approx. 28g (2 tbsps)
- Chili flakes: approx. 2.5g (1 tsp)
- Salt: approx. 5g (1 tsp)
- Water: approx. 180ml (¾ cup)

Directions:

- Spiralise the jicama with the help of a spiraliser and place the jicama spirals in the saucepan.
- Add butter, chili flakes, and salt.
- Then, add water and heat the ingredients until the butter is melted.
- Mix it up well.
- Close the lid and cook noodles for 4 minutes over a medium heat.
- Stir the jicama noodles well before transferring them to the serving plates.

Nutritients Per Serving: Calories: 182 kcal, Carbohydrates: 8.5 g, Protein: 6.8 g, Fat: 15.3 g, Sodium: 75 mg, Phosphorus: 110 mg, Potassium: 140 mg.

33. Mushroom Tacos

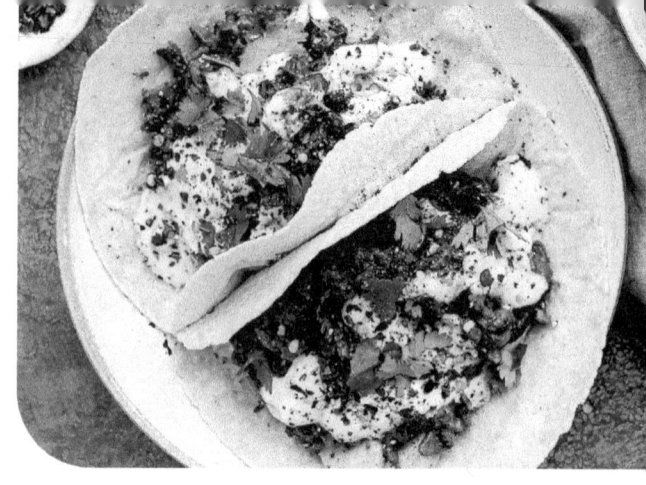

Servings: 6 **Preparation Time:** 10 minutes **Cooking Time:** 15 minutes

Ingredients:

- Spring greens
- Mushrooms, chopped: approx. 280g (2 cups)
- White onion, diced: approx. 150g (1 unit)
- Taco seasoning: approx. 8g (1 tbsp)
- Coconut oil: approx. 15ml (1 tbsp)
- Salt: approx. 2.5g (½ tsp)
- Fresh parsley: approx. 15g (¼ cup)
- Mayonnaise: approx. 15g (1 tbsp)

Directions:

- Melt the coconut oil in the skillet.
- Add the chopped mushrooms and diced onion, and stir.
- Close the lid and let it cook for 10 minutes.
- After this, sprinkle the taco seasoning over it. Add salt and the fresh parsley.
- Stir the mixture to ensure everything is coated in the seasonings and cook for 5 minutes more.
- Then add the mayonnaise and stir well.
- Chill the mushroom mixture a little.
- Fill the spring greens with the mushroom mixture and fold them.

Nutrients per Serving: Calories 18kcal, Fats 0.8mg, Carbs 2.8mg, Proteins 0.9g Phosphorus: 150mg, Sodium: 75mg, Potassium: 250mg.

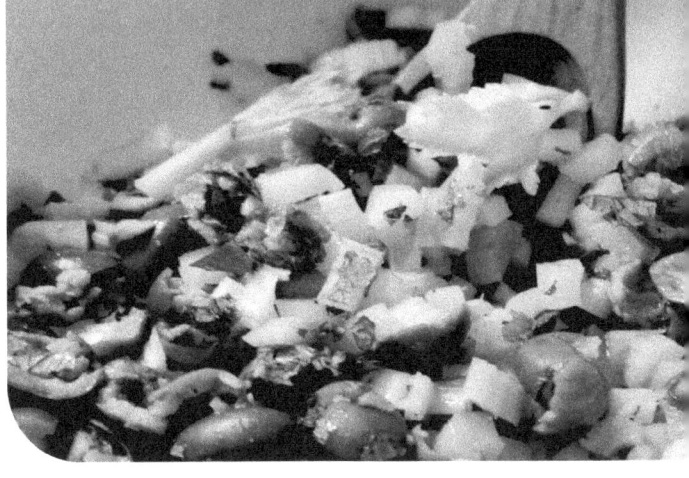

34. Minty Olives Salad

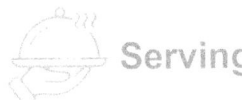 Servings: 4

 Preparation Time: 10 minutes

 Cooking Time: 0 minutes

Ingredients:

- 1 cup kalamata olives, pitted and sliced
- 1 cup black olives, pitted and halved
- 1 red onion, chopped
- 2 tablespoons oregano, chopped
- 1 tablespoon mint, chopped
- 2 tablespoons balsamic vinegar
- ¼ cup olive oil
- 2 teaspoons Italian herbs, dried
- A pinch of sea salt and black pepper

Directions:

- In a salad bowl, add and mix all of the ingredients and serve cold.

Nutrients per Serving: Calories: 240 kcal, Carbohydrate: 11.6 g, Protein: 12 g, Fat: 8.2 g, Sodium: 75 mg, Phosphorus: 110 mg, Potassium: 10 mg.

35. Bean and Cucumber Salad

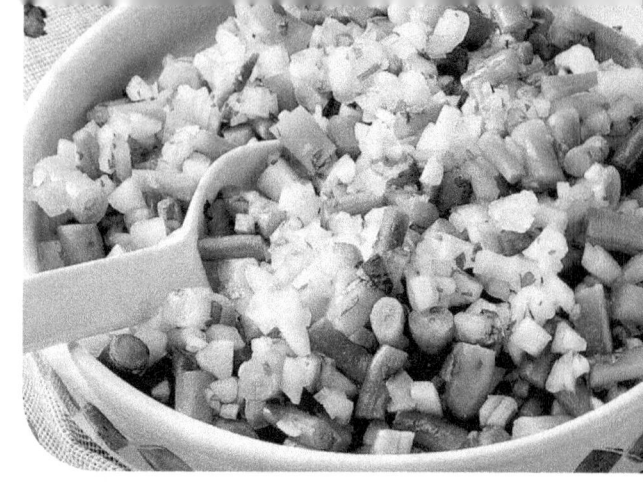

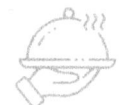 Servings: 4

 Preparation Time: 10 minutes

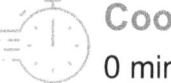 Cooking Time: 0 minutes

Ingredients:

- Canned great northern beans, drained and rinsed: approx. 280g (10 oz)
- Olive oil: approx. 30ml (2 tbsps)
- Baby rocket: approx. 25g (½ cup)
- Cucumber, sliced: approx. 120g (1 cup)
- Parsley, chopped: approx. 15g (1 tbsp)
- Sea salt and black pepper: to taste
- Balsamic vinegar: approx. 30ml (2 tbsps)

Directions:

- In a bowl, mix all of the ingredients and serve cold

Nutrients per Serving: Calories: 190 kcal, Carbohydrate: 11.6 g, Protein: 4.6 mg, Fat: 8.1 mg, Sodium: 75 mg, Phosphorus: 110 mg, Potassium: 200 mg.

Chapter no. 8

Fish And Seafood Recipes

You can still enjoy seafood while on renal diet. Here are some recipes.

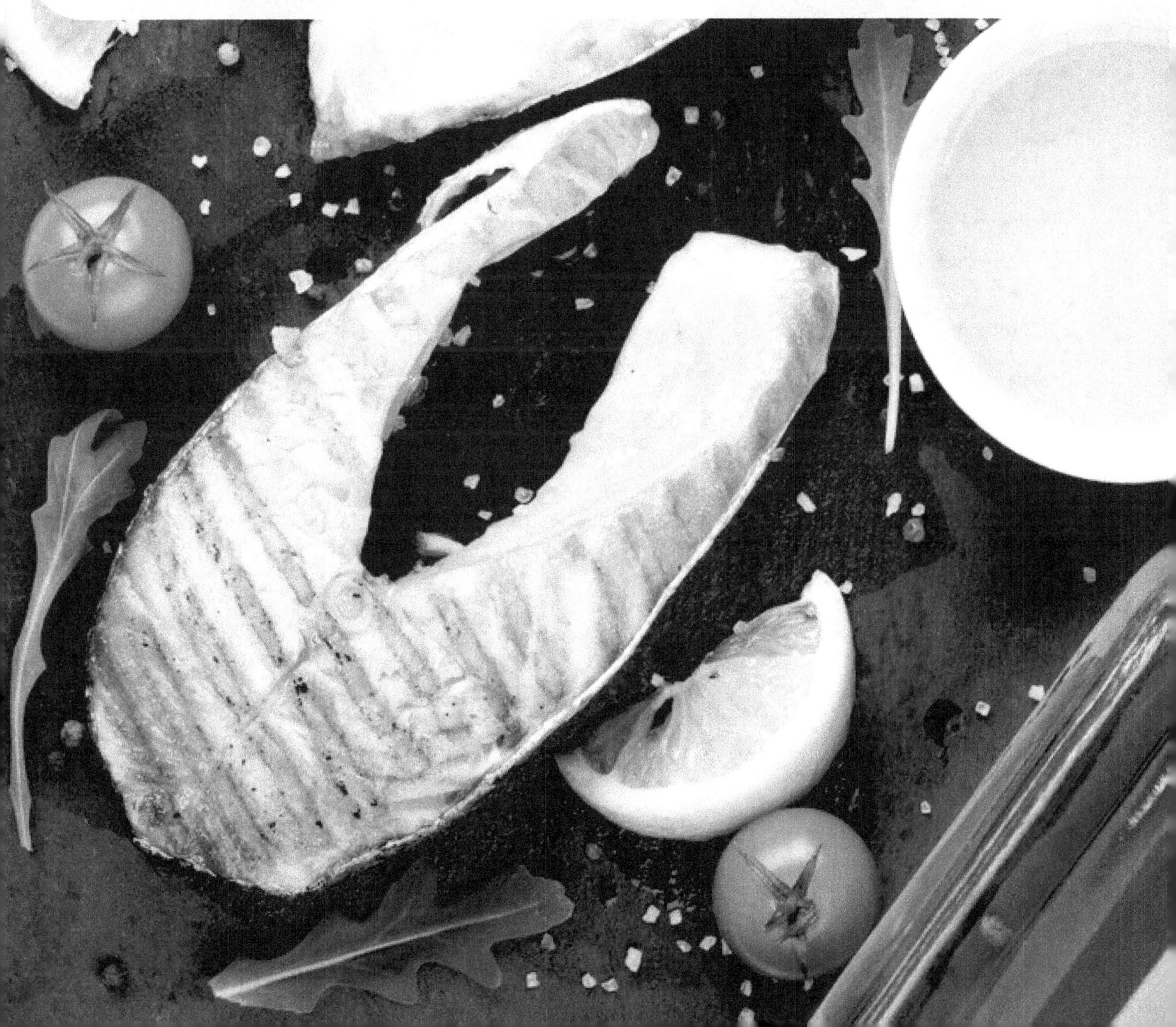

36. Baked sole with caramelized onion

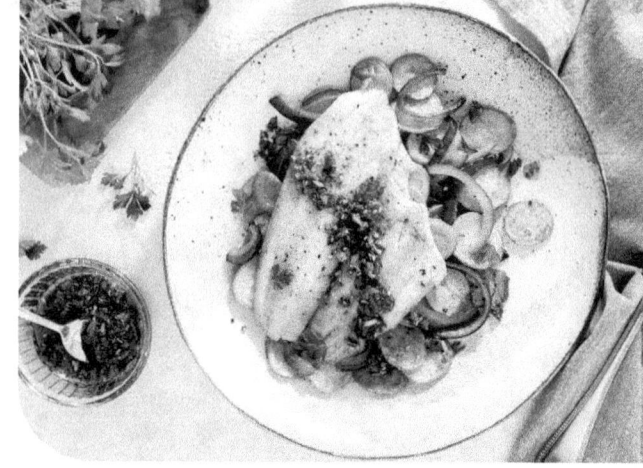

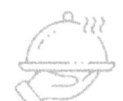 **Servings:** 4

 **Preparation Time:** 10 minutes

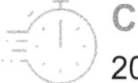 **Cooking Time:** 20 minutes

Ingredients:

- Onion, finely chopped: approx. 150g (1 cup)
- Low-sodium vegetable broth: approx. 120ml (½ cup)
- Yellow summer squash, sliced: approx. 120g (1 unit)
- Frozen broccoli florets: approx. 280g (2 cups)
- Sole fillets: 4 units, each approx. 85g (3 oz)
- Salt: to taste
- Olive oil: approx. 30ml (2 tbsps)
- Baking soda: a pinch
- Dried basil leaves: approx. 1g (1 tsp)

Directions:

- Preheat the oven to 218°C.
- Add the onions to a skillet. Cook for 1 minute. Then, stirring constantly, cook for another 4 minutes.
- Remove the onions from the heat.
- Pour the broth into a baking tray with a lip and arrange the squash and broccoli on the sheet in a single layer. Top the vegetables with the fish. Sprinkle salt on the fish and drizzle everything with olive oil.
- Bake the fish and the vegetables for 10 minutes.
- While the fish is baking, return the onions to the skillet and set the stove to a medium-high heat. Stir in a pinch of baking soda.
- Transfer the onions to a plate.
- Top the fish evenly with the onions. Sprinkle with the basil.
- Return the fish to the oven. Bake it for 8 to 10 minutes and serve the fish on the vegetables.

Nutrients per Serving: Calories: 188 kcal, Carbohydrate: 12 g, Protein: 21 g, Fat: 6 g, Sodium: 150 mg, Phosphorus: 150 mg, Potassium: 600 mg.

37. Thai tuna wraps

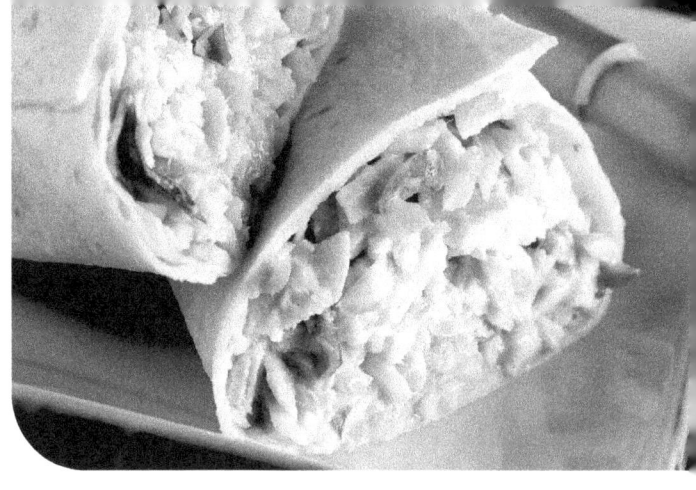

Servings: 4 **Preparation Time:** 10 minutes **Cooking Time:** 0-minute

Ingredients:

- Unsalted peanut butter: approx. 60g (¼ cup)
- Freshly squeezed lemon juice: approx. 30ml (2 tbsps)
- Low-sodium soy sauce: approx. 5ml (1 tsp)
- Ground ginger: approx. 1.5g (½ tsp)
- Cayenne pepper: approx. 0.3g (⅛ tsp)
- No-salt-added or low-sodium tuna chunks, drained: 1 can (approx. 170g or 6 oz)
- Red cabbage, shredded: approx. 70g (1 cup)
- Spring onions, white and green parts, chopped: approx. 30g (2 spring onions)
- Carrots, grated: approx. 110g (1 cup)
- Butter lettuce leaves: 8 leaves

Directions:

- In a medium-sized bowl, stir the peanut butter, lemon juice, soy sauce, ginger, and cayenne pepper until well combined.
- Stir in the tuna, cabbage, spring onions, and carrots.
- Divide the tuna filling evenly between the butter lettuce leaves and serve

Nutrients per Serving: Calories: 202 kcal, Carbohydrate: 10g, Protein: 16 g, Fat: 11 g, Sodium: 320 mg, Phosphorus: 331 mg, Potassium: 150 mg

38. Grilled fish and vegetable packets

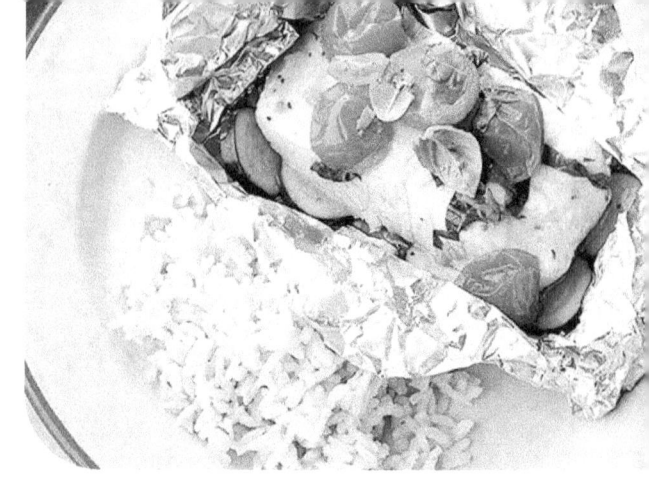

 Servings: 4

 Preparation Time: 15 minutes

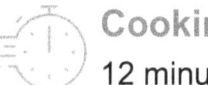 Cooking Time: 12 minutes

Ingredients:

- Mushrooms, sliced: approx. 225g (1 unit, 8 oz)
- Leek, white and green parts, chopped: approx. 100g (1 unit)
- Frozen corn: approx. 160g (1 cup)
- Atlantic cod fillets: 4 units, each approx. 115g (4 oz)
- Juice of 1 lemon
- Olive oil: approx. 45ml (3 tbsps)

Directions:

- Prepare the outdoor grill by lighting some medium-sized coals and set the grill 6 inches away from the coals.
- Tear off four 30-inch strips of heavy-duty aluminium foil.
- Arrange the mushrooms, leek, and corn in the centre of each piece of foil and top with the fish.
- Drizzle the fish and vegetables evenly with the lemon juice and olive oil.
- Bring the longer sides of the foil together at the top and, holding the edges together, fold them over twice and then fold in the shorter sides to form a sealed parcel with room for the steam.
- Put the parcels on the grill for 10 to 12 minutes until the vegetables are tender but still crisp and the fish flakes when tested with a fork. Be careful opening the parcels because the escaping steam can scald.

Nutrients per Serving: Calories: 175 kcal, Carbohydrate: 8 g, Protein: 17 g, Fat: 10 g, Sodium: 98 mg, Phosphorus: 153 mg; Potassium: 400 mg.

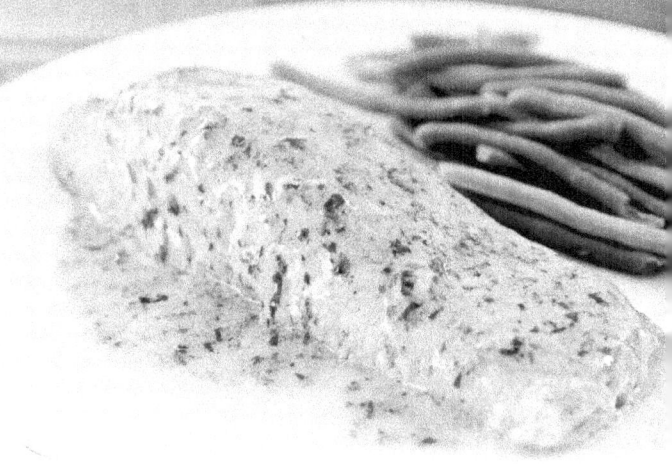

39. Lemon butter salmon

 **Servings:** 6

 **Preparation Time:** 15 minutes

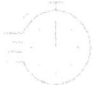 **Cooking Time:** 15 minutes

Ingredients:

- Butter: approx. 15g (1 tbsp)
- Olive oil: approx. 30ml (2 tbsps)
- Dijon mustard: approx. 15g (1 tbsp)
- Lemon juice: approx. 15ml (1 tbsp)
- Garlic cloves, crushed: 2 units
- Dried dill: approx. 1g (1 tsp)
- Dried basil leaves: approx. 1g (1 tsp)
- Capers: approx. 15g (1 tbsp)
- Salmon filet: approx. 680g (24 oz)

Directions:

- Put all ingredients except the salmon in a saucepan over a medium heat.
- Bring to a boil and then simmer for 5 minutes.
- Preheat your grill.
- Create a parcel using foil.
- Place the sauce and salmon inside.
- Seal the parcel.
- Grill for 12 minutes

Nutrients per Serving: Calories: 117 kcal, Carbohydrate: 5.4 g, Protein: 8.1 g, Fat: 7.2 g, Sodium: 180 mg, Phosphorus: 111 mg, Potassium: 400mg

40. Shrimp & broccoli

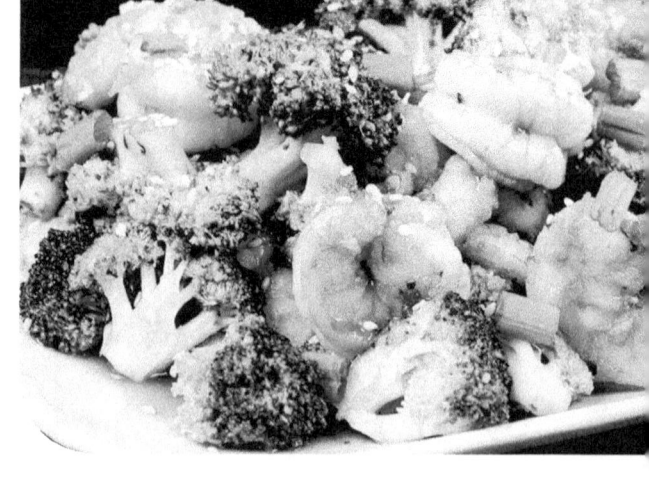

Servings: 4

Preparation Time: 10 minutes

Cooking Time: 5 minutes

Ingredients:

- Olive oil: approx. 15ml (1 tbsp)
- Garlic clove, minced: 1 unit
- Shrimp: approx. 454g (1 lb)
- Red sweet pepper: approx. 30g (¼ cup)
- Broccoli florets, steamed: approx. 140g (1 cup)
- Cream cheese: approx. 280g (10 oz)
- Garlic powder: approx. 1.5g (½ tsp)
- Lemon juice: approx. 60ml (¼ cup)
- Ground peppercorns: approx. 2g (¾ tsp)
- Single cream: approx. 60ml (¼ cup)

Directions:

- Pour the oil into a pan and cook garlic for 30 seconds.
- Add shrimp and cook for 2 minutes.
- Add the rest of the ingredients.
- Mix well and cook for 2 minutes.

Nutrients per Serving: Calories: 383 kcal, Carbohydrate: 46 g, Protein: 24 g, Fat: 11 g, Sodium: 253 mg, Phosphorus: 266 mg, Potassium: 275 mg.

41. Shrimp in garlic sauce

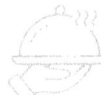 **Preparation Time:** 10 minutes    **Cooking Time:** 6 minutes   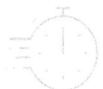 **Servings:** 4

Ingredients:

- Butter (unsalted): approx. 45g (3 tbsps)
- Onion, minced: approx. 60g (¼ cup)
- Garlic cloves, minced: 3 units
- Shrimp, shelled and deveined: approx. 454g (1 lb)
- Single cream: approx. 120ml (½ cup)
- White wine: approx. 60ml (¼ cup)
- Fresh basil: approx. 8g (2 tbsps)
- Black pepper: to taste

Directions:

- Add butter to a pan over a medium-low heat. Let it melt.
- Add the onion and garlic. Cook it for 1-2 minutes.
- Add the shrimp and cook for 2 minutes.
- Transfer the shrimp to a serving platter and set aside.
- Add the rest of the ingredients. Simmer for 3 minutes.
- Pour sauce over the shrimp and serve.

Nutrients per Serving: Calories: 469 kcal, Carbohydrate: 28 g, Protein: 28 g, Fat: 28 g, Sodium: 300 mg, Phosphorus: 260 mg, Potassium: 260 mg

42. Fish taco

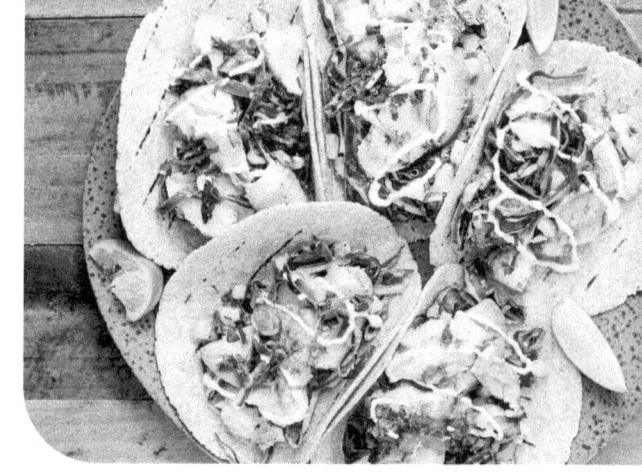

Servings: 6

Preparation Time: 40 minutes

Cooking Time: 10 minutes

Ingredients:

- Lime juice: approx. 15ml (1 tbsp)
- Olive oil: approx. 15ml (1 tbsp)
- Garlic clove, minced: 1 unit
- Cod fillets: approx. 454g (1 lb)
- Ground cumin: approx. 2.5g (½ tsp)
- Black pepper: a pinch
- Chili powder: approx. 1.5g (½ tsp)
- Sour cream: approx. 60ml (¼ cup)
- Mayonnaise: approx. 120ml (½ cup)
- Non-dairy milk: approx. 30ml (2 tbsps)
- Cabbage, shredded: approx. 90g (1 cup)
- Onion, chopped: approx. 60g (½ cup)
- Coriander, chopped: approx. 15g (½ bunch)
- Corn tortillas: 12 units

Directions:

- Drizzle lemon juice over the fish fillet.
- Coat it with olive oil and then season with garlic, cumin, pepper and chili powder.
- Let it marinate for 30 minutes.
- Broil fish for 10 minutes, flipping halfway through.
- Flake the fish using a fork.
- In a bowl, mix sour cream, milk and mayonnaise.
- Assemble tacos by filling each tortilla with the mayonnaise mixture, cabbage, onion, coriander and fish flakes

Nutrients per Serving: Calories: 482 kcal, Carbohydrate: 46 g, Protein: 33 g, Fat: 11 g, Sodium: 70 mg, Phosphorus: 50 mg, Potassium: 33 mg.

Chapter no. 9

Renal-Friendly Meat Options

People with impaired kidney function must follow a suitable diet to reduce the quantity of waste in their blood. Waste in the blood is a result of consumed food and drinks. A renal diet may improve kidney function and delay the onset of total kidney failure. This diet is frequently advised for individuals with end-stage or late-stage CKD. It is defined by a decrease in sodium, potassium, and phosphor in the diet. Certain limits are in place to avoid accumulating these micronutrients in the bloodstream and to minimise problems, including hypertension, fluid overload, arrhythmia, ortho diseases, and vascular calcifications. The following chapter contains meat-based recipes while on a renal diet.

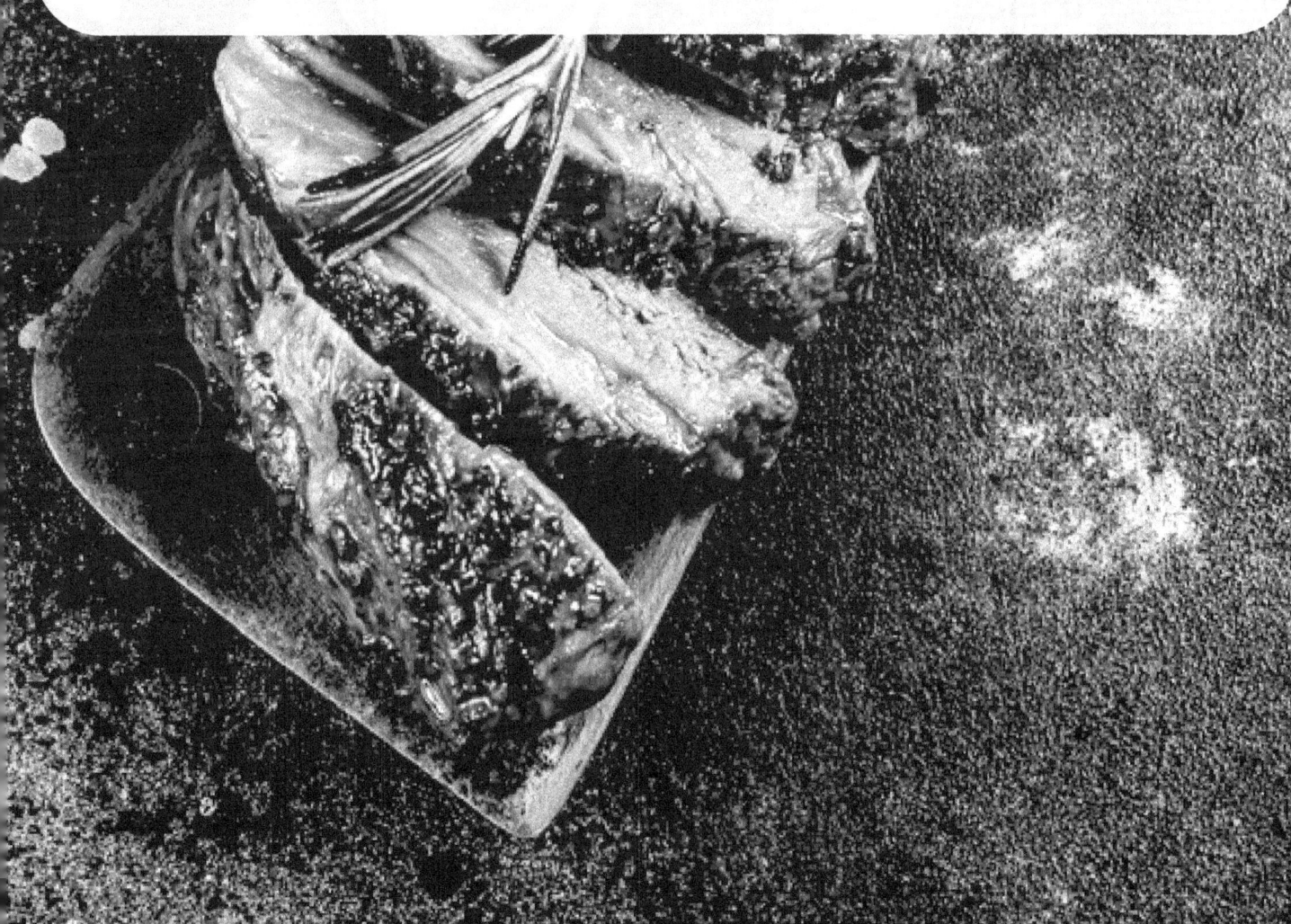

43. Pork loins with leeks

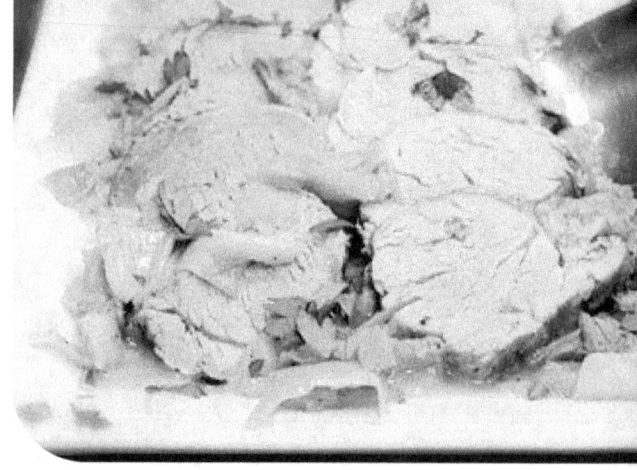

Servings: 2

Preparation Time: 10 minutes

Cooking Time: 35 minutes

Ingredients:

- Sliced leek: approx. 90g (1 unit)
- Mustard seeds: approx. 15g (1 tbsp)
- Pork tenderloin: approx. 170g (6 oz)
- Cumin seeds: approx. 15g (1 tbsp)
- Dry mustard: approx. 5g (1 tbsp)
- Extra virgin olive oil: approx. 15ml (1 tbsp)

Directions:

- Heat the grill to a medium-high heat.
- In a dry skillet, heat the mustard and cumin seeds until they start to pop (3-5 minutes).
- Grind seeds using a pestle and mortar or spice blender, then mix in the dry mustard.
- Coat the pork on both sides with the mustard blend and add to a baking tray to grill for 25-30 minutes or until cooked through. Turn once halfway through.
- Remove and place to one side.
- Heat the oil in a pan on medium heat and add the leeks for 5-6 minutes or until soft.
- Serve the pork tenderloin on a bed of leeks and enjoy.

Nutrients per Serving: Calories: 306 kcal, Carbohydrate: 10 g, Protein: 23 g, Fat: 20 g, Sodium: 86 mg, Phosphorus: 269 mg, Potassium: 450 mg.

44. Chinese beef wraps

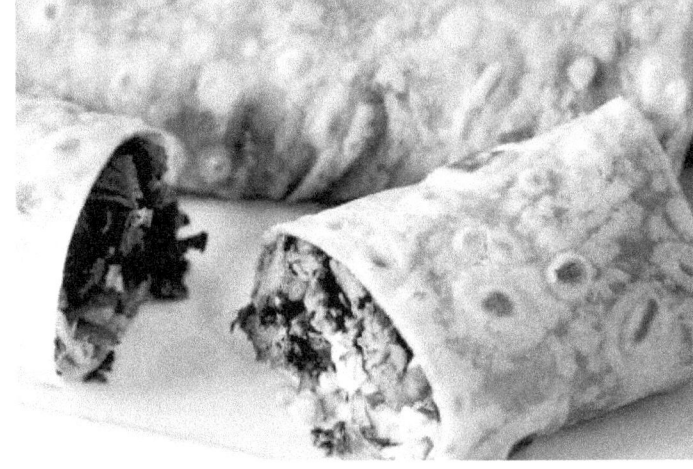

 **Servings:** 2

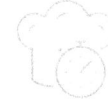 **Preparation Time:** 10 minutes

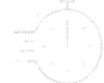 **Cooking Time:** 30 minutes

Ingredients:

- Iceberg lettuce leaves: 2 leaves
- Cucumber, diced: approx. 75g (½ cup)
- Canola oil: approx. 5ml (1 tsp)
- Lean ground beef: approx. 140g (5 oz)
- Ground ginger: approx. 2g (1 tsp)
- Chili flakes: approx. 5g (1 tbsp)
- Garlic clove, minced: 1 unit
- Rice wine vinegar: approx. 15ml (1 tbsp)

Directions:

- Mix the ground meat with garlic, rice wine vinegar, chili flakes and ginger in a bowl.
- Heat oil in a skillet over medium heat.
- Add the beef to the pan and cook for 20-25 minutes or until cooked.
- Serve beef mixture with diced cucumber in each lettuce wrap and fold

Nutrients per Serving: Calories: 139 kcal, Carbohydrate: 2 g, Protein: 18 g, Fat: 5 g, Sodium: 150 mg, Phosphorus: 278 mg, Potassium: 250 mg.

45. Grilled skirt steak

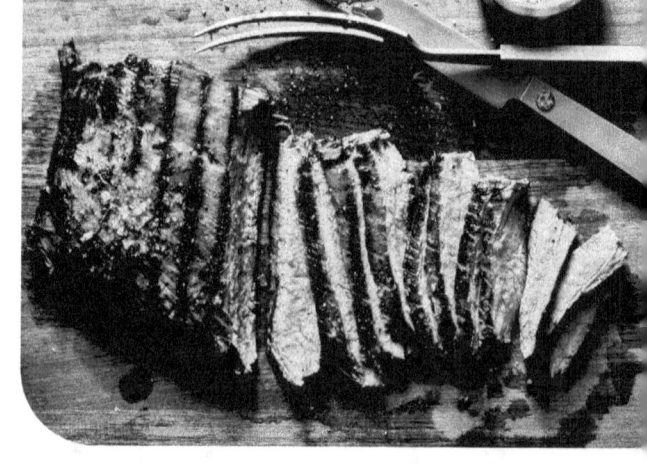

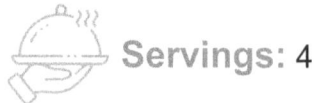 **Servings:** 4

 **Preparation Time:** 15 minutes

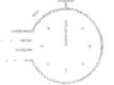 **Cooking Time:** 8-9 minutes

Ingredients:

- Fresh ginger herb, grated finely: approx. 10g (2 tsps)
- Fresh lime zest, grated finely: approx. 10g (2 tsps)
- Coconut sugar: approx. 50g (¼ cup)
- Fish sauce: approx. 10ml (2 tsps)
- Fresh lime juice: approx. 30ml (2 tbsps)
- Coconut milk: approx. 120ml (½ cup)
- Beef skirt steak, trimmed and cut into 4-inch slices lengthwise: approx. 454g (1 lb)
- Salt: to taste

Directions:

- In a large sealable bag, mix all the ingredients except the steak and salt.
- Add the steak and generously coat with the marinade.
- Seal the bag and refrigerate to marinate for about 4-12 hours.
- Preheat the grill to high heat. Grease the grill grate.
- Remove the steak from the refrigerator and discard the marinade.
- With a paper towel, dry the steak and sprinkle with salt evenly.
- Place the steak on the grill and cook it for approximately 3 ½ minutes.
- Flip it and cook for around 2 ½-5 minutes or till it has reached the desired doneness.
- Remove from grill and keep aside for approximately 5 minutes before slicing.
- With a sharp knife, cut into slices and serve

Nutrients per Serving: Calories: 156 kcal, Carbohydrate: 4 g, Protein: 14 g, Fat: 2 g, Sodium: 250 mg, Phosphorus: 150 mg, Potassium: 200 mg

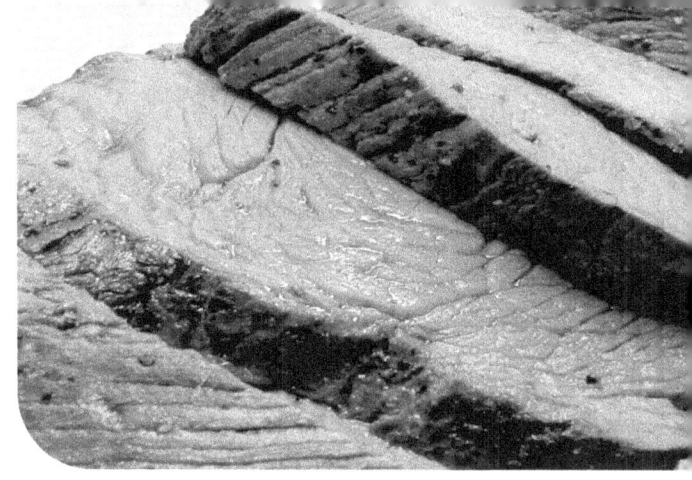

46. Roast beef

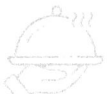 **Preparation Time:** 25 minutes

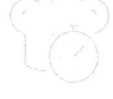 **Cooking Time:** 55 minutes

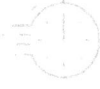 **Servings:** 1

Ingredients:

- 100 g quality beef, rump or sirloin tip

Direction:

- Place the beef in roasting pan on a shallow rack.
- Season with pepper and herbs.
- Insert a meat thermometer in the centre or thickest part of the beef.
- Roast to the desired degree of doneness.
- After removing it from the oven, let it rest for about 15 minutes.
- In the end, the roast should be moister than well done

Nutrients per Serving: Calories: 393 kcal, Carbohydrate: 10 g, Protein: 36 g, Fat: 12 g, Sodium: 70 g, Phosphorus: 200 mg, Potassium: 100 mg.

47. Beef brochettes

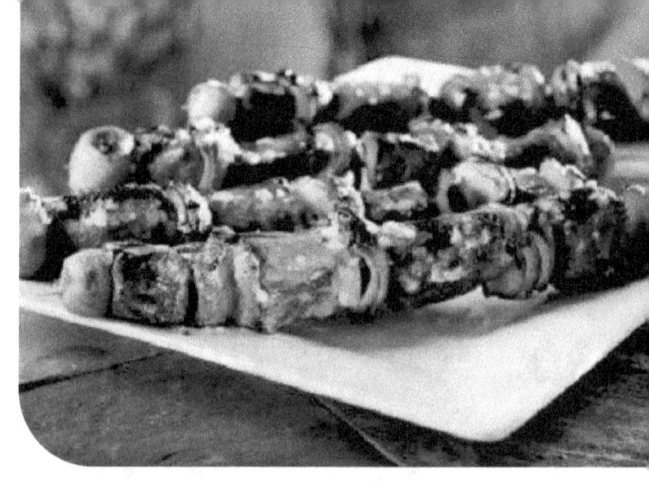

Servings: 1

Preparation Time: 20 minutes

Cooking Time: 1 hour

Ingredients:

- Large onion, sliced: approx. 225g (1 unit)
- Thick steak: approx. 907g (2 lbs)
- Medium sweet pepper, sliced: approx. 120g (1 unit)
- Bay leaf: 1 unit
- Vegetable oil: approx. 60ml (¼ cup)
- Lemon juice: approx. 120ml (½ cup)
- Garlic cloves, crushed: 2 units

Directions:

- Dice the beef and place them into a plastic bag.
- Mix the marinade ingredients in a small bowl.
- Pour over the beef in the bag.
- Seal the bag and chill for 3 to 5 hours.
- Separate the onion, beef, green pepper and pineapple.
- Grill for about 9 minutes on each side

Nutrients per Serving: Calories: 158 kcal, Carbohydrates: 0 g, Protein: 24 g, Fats 6 g, Sodium: 10 mg, Phosphorus: 30 mg, Potassium: 460 mg

48. Country fried steak

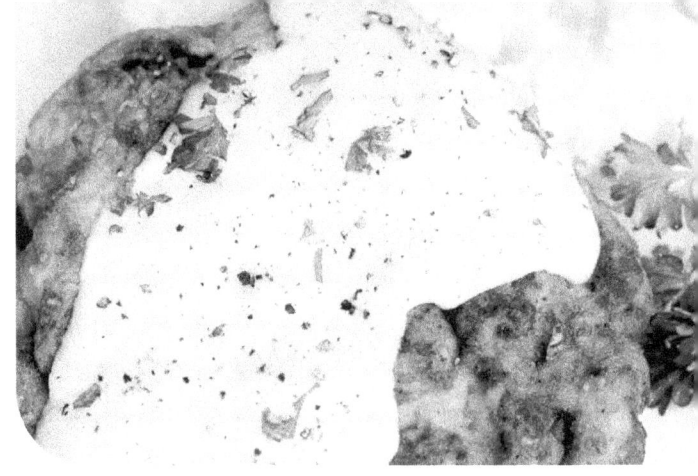

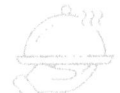 Servings: 3

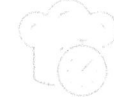 Preparation Time: 10 minutes

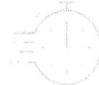 Cooking Time: 1 hour and 40 minutes

Ingredients:

- Large onion: approx. 225g (1 unit)
- Flour: approx. 60g (½ cup)
- Vegetable oil: approx. 45ml (3 tbsps)
- Pepper: a pinch
- Rump steak: approx. 680g (1.5 lbs)
- Paprika: approx. 2.5g (½ tsp)
- Water: approx. 150ml

Directions:

- Trim excess fat from the steak.
- Cut the steak into small pieces.
- Combine flour, paprika and pepper and mix.
- Preheat the skillet and add oil.
- Cook steak on all sides.
- When the colour of the steak is brown, move it to a platter.
- Add water to the skillet and stir it.
- Return the seared steak to skillet. If necessary, add water again so that the steak does not stick

Nutrients per Serving: Calories: 304 kcal, Carbohydrate: 11 g, Protein: 35 g, Fat: 15 g, Sodium: 30 mg, Phosphorus: 70 mg, Potassium: 200 mg

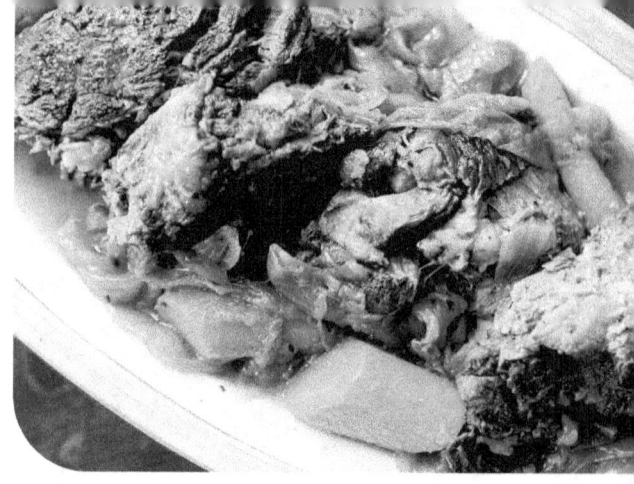

49. Beef pot roast

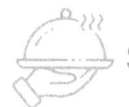 **Servings:** 3

 **Preparation Time:** 20 minutes

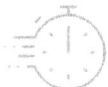 **Cooking Time:** 1 hour

Ingredients:

- Round bone beef
- Chuck beef: approx. 907g - 1814g (2-4 lbs)

Direction:

- Trim off excess fat.
- Place a tablespoon of oil in a large skillet over a medium heat.
- Roll beef in flour and brown on all sides in the skillet.
- After the meat gets has been seared, reduce the heat to low.
- Season with pepper and herbs and add a ½ cup of water.
- Cook slowly for 1½ hours or until it looks ready

Nutrients per Serving: Calories: 248 kcal, Carbohydrate: 5 g, Protein: 30 g, Fat: 10 g, Sodium: 60 mg, Phosphorus: 190 mg

50. Homemade burgers

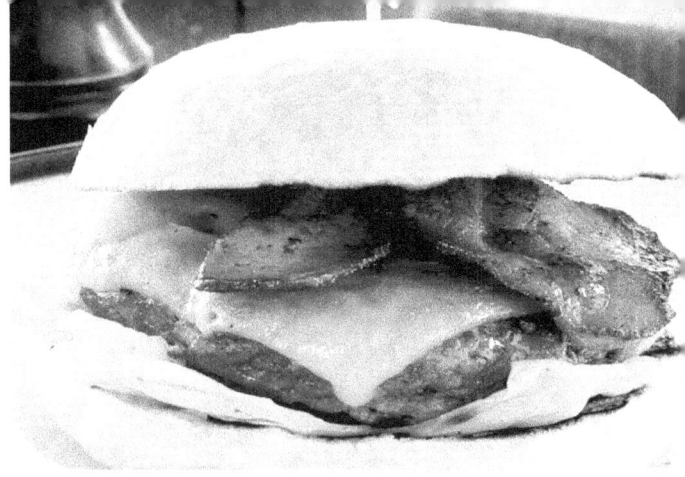

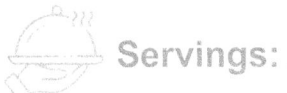 Servings: 2

 Preparation Time: 10 minutes

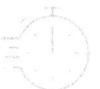 Cooking Time: 20 minutes

Ingredients:

- Lean ground beef: approx. 113g (4 oz)
- Black pepper: approx. 2.5g (1 tsp)
- Garlic clove, minced: 1 unit
- Olive oil: approx. 5ml (1 tsp)
- Onion, finely diced: approx. 30g (¼ cup)
- Balsamic vinegar: approx. 15ml (1 tbsp)
- Brie cheese, crumbled: approx. 14g (½ oz)
- Mustard: approx. 5g (1 tsp)

Directions:

- Season the ground beef with pepper and then mix in the minced garlic.
- Form burger shapes with the ground beef using the palms of your hands.
- Heat a skillet on medium to high heat, and then add the oil.
- Sauté the onions for 5-10 minutes until browned.
- Then add the balsamic vinegar to the onions and sauté for another 5 minutes.
- Remove and set aside.
- Add the burgers to the pan and cook on the same heat for 5-6 minutes before flipping and heating for 5-6 minutes until cooked through.
- Spread the mustard onto each burger.
- Crumble the brie cheese over each burger and serve!
- Try with a crunchy side salad!
- *Tip:* if using fresh beef and not defrosted, prepare double the ingredients and freeze the burgers in clingfilm (after cooling) for up to 1 month.
- Thoroughly defrost before cooking it in the oven. Ensure it is completely cooked before it is served

Nutrients per Serving: Calories: 157 kcal, Carbohydrate: 0 g, Protein: 24 g, Fat: 13 g, Sodium: 150 mg, Phosphorus: 204 mg, Potassium: 130 mg.

51. Peppercorn Pork Chops

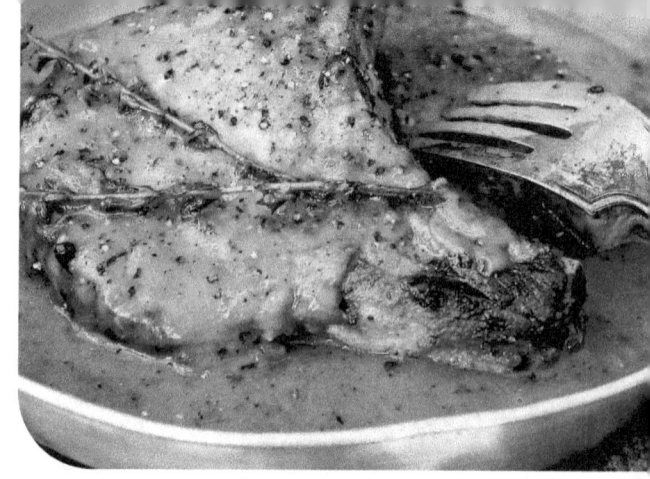

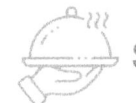 **Servings:** 4

 **Preparation Time:** 30 min

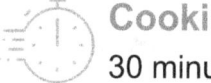 **Cooking Time:** 30 minutes

Ingredients:

- Black peppercorns, crushed: approx. 15g (1 tbsp)
- Pork loin chops: The quantity varies depending on the desired serving size.
- Olive oil: approx. 30ml (2 tbsps)
- Butter: approx. 60g (¼ cup)
- Garlic cloves: The quantity depends on personal preference.
- Green and red sweet peppers: approx. 120g (1 cup)
- Pineapple juice: approx. 120ml (½ cup)

Directions:

- Sprinkle and press the peppercorns into both sides of the pork chops.
- Dice the sweet peppers.
- Heat the oil, butter and garlic cloves in a large skillet over a medium heat, stirring frequently.
- Add the pork chops and cook uncovered for 5–6 minutes.
- Add the sweet peppers and pineapple juice to the pork chops.
- Cover and simmer for another 5–6 minutes or until pork is thoroughly cooked.

Nutrition: Calories: 317 kcal, Carbohydrate: 9.2 g, Protein: 13.2 g, Fat: 25.7 g, Sodium: 126 mg, Phosphorus: 115 mg, Potassium: 250 mg.

52. Pork Chops with Apples and Onions

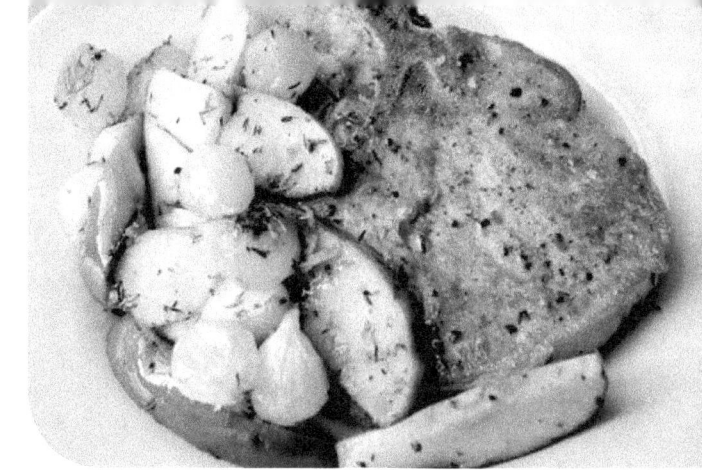

Servings: 4   **Preparation Time:** 30 min   **Cooking Time:** 60 minutes

Ingredients:

- Pork chops: The quantity varies depending on the desired serving size.
- Salt and pepper: to taste
- Onions, sliced into rings: 2 units
- Apples, peeled, cored, and sliced into rings: 2 units
- Honey: The quantity is missing. Please specify.
- Freshly ground black pepper: approx. 10g (2 tsps)

Directions:

- Pork chops: The quantity varies depending on the desired serving size.
- Salt and pepper: to taste
- Onions, sliced into rings: 2 units
- Apples, peeled, cored, and sliced into rings: 2 units
- Honey: The quantity is missing. Please specify.
- Freshly ground black pepper: approx. 10g (2 tsps)

Nutrition: Calories: 307 kcal, Carbohydrate: 26.8 g, Protein: 15.1 g, Fat: 16.1 g, Sodium: 100 mg, Phosphorus: 200 mg, Potassium: 250 mg.

53. Baked Lamb Chops

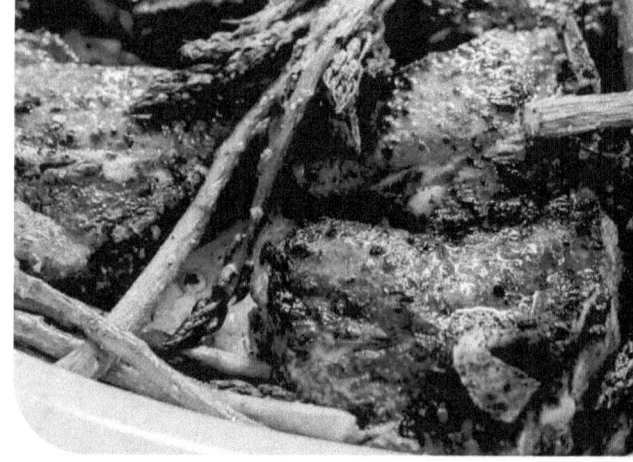

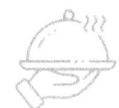 Servings: 4

 Preparation Time: 10 min

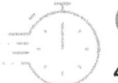 Cooking Time: 45 minutes

Ingredients:

- 2 eggs
- Worcestershire sauce: approx. 10ml (2 tsps)
- Lamb chops: 8 units, each approx. 155g
- Graham crackers: approx. 200g (2 cups)

Directions:

- Preheat the oven to 190°C.
- Mix the eggs and Worcestershire sauce in a medium bowl. Stir well.
- Dip each lamb chop in the sauce and lightly dredge in the graham crackers. Then arrange them in a 9-inch-by-13-inch baking dish.
- Bake at 190°C for 20 minutes. Turn the chops over and cook for 20 more minutes.

Nutrition: Calories: 176 kcal, Carbohydrate: 21.9 g, Protein: 9.1 g, Fat 5.7 g, Sodium: 150 mg, Phosphorus: 100 mg, Potassium: 150 mg.

54. Grilled Lamb Chops with Pineapple

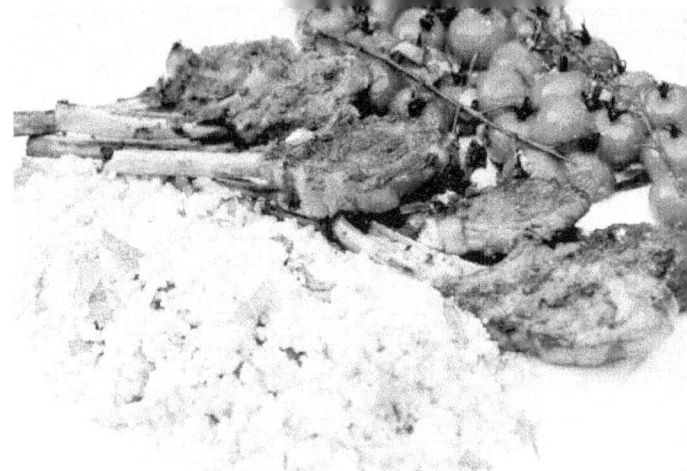

Servings: 4

Preparation Time: 15 min

Cooking Time: 55 minutes

Ingredients:

- 1 lemon, zest and juiced
- Fresh oregano, chopped: approx. 8g (2 tbsps)
- 2 garlic cloves, minced
- Black pepper: to taste
- Lamb chops: 8 units, each approx. 85g
- Fresh unsweetened pineapple juice: approx. 120ml (½ cup)
- Pineapples: approx. 160g (1 cup)

Directions:

- Whisk together the lemon zest and juice, oregano, garlic, salt, and black pepper in a bowl.
- Pour into a resealable plastic bag.
- Add the lamb chops, coat with the marinade, squeeze out excess air, and seal the bag. Set aside to marinate.
- Preheat an outdoor grill to a medium-high heat, and lightly oil the grate.
- Pour the pineapple juice into a small saucepan over a high heat.
- Reduce the heat to medium-low and continue simmering until the liquid has reduced to half its original volume. It should take about 45 minutes.
- Stir in the pineapples and set aside.
- Remove the lamb from the marinade and shake off the excess. Discard the remaining marinade.
- Cook the chops on the grill until they start to firm and are reddish-pink and juicy in the centre. This is about 4 minutes per side to reach medium rare. Serve the chops drizzled with the pineapple reduction.

Nutrition: Calories: 69 kcal, Carbohydrate: 8.5 g, Protein: 5.9 g, Fat: 1.6 g, Sodium: 45 mg, Phosphorus: 65 mg, Potassium: 200 mg

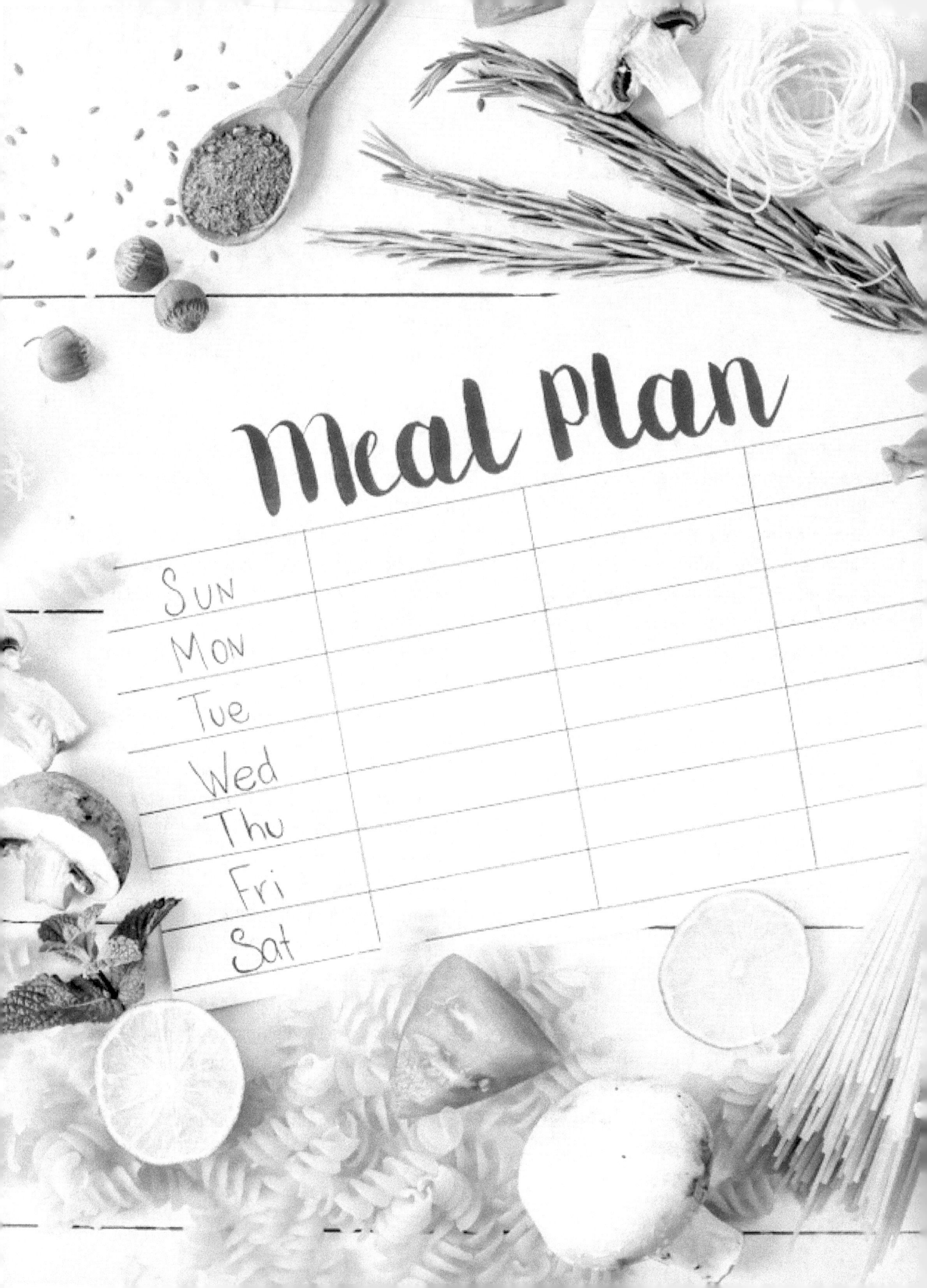

Chapter no. 10

28 Days Meal Plan

DAY 1

Breakfast

- 1 serving of chocolate smoothie, with 1 tablespoon of peanut butter, either mixed in or separate
- 1 slice of 100% wholewheat bread with 1 tablespoon of goat cheese and coffee with up to 200gr of non-fat milk

Lunch

- 1 serving of glazed snap peas
- ½ cup cherry tomatoes
- ½ cup baby carrots
- 1 medium apple

Snack

- 200gr of non-fat plain yoghurt
- 1 medium apple
- 10 almonds

Dinner

- 1 serving of baked aubergine slices
- 1 serving crack slaw
- 4 small roasted red potatoes
- 2 healthy berry oatmeal muffins with apple and blueberry crumble

DAY 2

Breakfast

- 2 slices of toast with almond butter and banana
- 200 gr of non-fat milk or coffee with up to 200 gr of non-fat milk

Lunch

- 2 servings of salad with vinaigrette
- ½ of a sliced avocado
- 10 almonds
- 1 medium peach

Snack

- 1 medium apple, sliced, with 1 tablespoon of almond butter

Dinner

- 1 serving of stuffed sweet peppers
- 1 cup of steamed broccoli
- 1 serving of lemon parfait or 1 serving of berry sundae

DAY 3

Breakfast
- 1 hard-boiled egg and 1 serving of apple oatmeal custard
- 200 gr of non-fat milk

Lunch
- 1 serving of curried chicken salad pitta sandwich
- 1 cup of baby carrots and sliced sweet peppers
- 1 cup of cherries

SNACK
- 200 gr of non-fat plain yoghurt
- 1 cup of mixed berries
- 20 almonds

DINNER
- 2 servings of roasted butternut squash soup, topped with 1 tablespoon of low-fat yoghurt
- 1 serving of Brussel sprout casserole
- 1 serving of chicken and mandarin salad
- 1 delicious orange and cinnamon biscotti

DAY 4

BREAKFAST
- 1 serving of quick and easy apple oatmeal custard

LUNCH
- 1 serving of grilled romaine salad with 1 tablespoon
- 100gr of roasted, boneless, skinless chicken breast
- ½ of a 100% wholewheat pitta bread
- 1 apple

SNACK
- ½ cup of non-fat cottage cheese with a ½ cup of sliced cucumbers and cherry tomatoes
- 1 medium orange

DINNER
- 1 serving of lemon butter salmon
- 1 cup of baked sweet potato
- 1 cup of steamed spinach

DAY 5

BREAKFAST
- 1 serving of tropical smoothie
- 2 simply baked pancakes
- 2 tablespoons of peanut butter or almond butter

LUNCH
- 1 serving of Italian veggie pitta with 100gr of grilled or roasted beef
- 200 gr of non-fat milk
- ½ cup of grapes

SNACK
- ¼ cup of hummus with sliced sweet pepper and cucumber

DINNER

- 1 homemade burger
- 1 serving of beans and cucumber salad
- 1 cup of boiled brown rice and courgette brownies

DAY 6

BREAKFAST

- 2 simple pancakes
- 2 tablespoons of real maple syrup
- Coffee with up to 200 gr of non-fat milk
- ½ cup of sliced strawberries

LUNCH

- 1 serving of turkey salad with 1 ½ cups of spinach
- 1 medium kiwi

SNACK

- 1 serving of chocolate smoothie

DINNER

- 1 serving of grilled skirt steak and a ¼ cup of grandma's guacamole (2 tablespoons)
- ½ cup of Anna's black beans
- 1 cup of pear and brie salad

DAY 7

BREAKFAST

- 1 serving of egg and sausage breakfast sandwich
- 1 tablespoon of almonds
- Coffee with 100gr of non-fat milk

LUNCH

- 1 serving of kale vegetable soup
- 200gr of non-fat milk
- 1 toasted cheese sandwich with reduced-fat mozzarella
- Cheese on 1 slice of 100% wholewheat bread (no sandwich)

SNACK

- 2 to 3 addictive cookies
- ½ cup of grapes

DINNER

- 2 slices of Mexican pizza
- 1 serving of pasta salad
- 1 serving of saskatoon berry pudding

DAY 8

BREAKFAST

- 2 egg whites only
- Coffee with up to 200gr of non-fat milk
- 1 slice of 100% wholewheat bread
- ½ cup of grapes

LUNCH

- 1 serving of chicken and mandarin salad
- ½ cup of baby carrots
- 1 medium peach

SNACK

- 20 almonds and an apple

DINNER

- 1 serving of coriander chili burgers
- ½ cup of rice
- 1 cup of steamed spinach

DAY 9

BREAKFAST

- Veggie omelette
- ½ cup of mixed berries
- Coffee with up to 200grfof non-fat milk

LUNCH

- 2 servings of chicken pasta salad
- 1 cup of sliced carrot, sweet pepper, and cucumber with 2 tablespoons of basic vinaigrette
- 1 medium pear

SNACK

- 100gr of non-fat cottage cheese
- ¼ cup of raw unsalted cashews
- 1 medium sliced apple

DINNER

- 1 serving of chow mein
- 1 serving of grilled asparagus
- 1 cup of brown rice
- 1 serving of raspberry cheesecake mousse

DAY 10

BREAKFAST

- 1 serving of egg with smashed avocado toast
- Coffee with up to 200gr of non-fat milk

LUNCH

- 1 serving of pasta salad
- 1 100% wholewheat pitta bread
- 1 medium peach

SNACK

- 1 serving of crunchy apple-maple snack mix
- baby carrots and sliced sweet pepper

DINNER

- 1 serving of baked, sunflower-seed-encrusted turkey cutlets
- 1 serving of lime and chickpea salad
- 1 medium baked sweet potato with 1 tablespoon of butter
- 1 serving of minty olive salad

DAY 11

BREAKFAST

- 1 serving of Wakeup Call! smoothie
- 1 hard-boiled egg
- 1 slice of 100% wholewheat toast

LUNCH

- 2 beef tacos
- Barley blueberry salad
- 1 medium orange

SNACK

- 1 100% wholewheat English muffin
- 2 tablespoons of peanut butter or almond butter and 1 apple

DINNER

- 1 serving of beef pot roast
- 1 ½ cups of white fish soup
- 1 cup of boiled brown rice
- 1 cup of frozen grapes

DAY 12

BREAKFAST

- 1 hardboiled egg
- 2 cheese and asparagus crêpe rolls with parsley
- Coffee with up to 200gr of non-fat milk

LUNCH

- 1 serving of roasted butternut squash soup
- ½ cup of sliced strawberries
- 1 cup of baby carrots

SNACK

- 200 gr of non-fat plain yoghurt
- ½ cup of blueberries
- ¼ cup of almonds

DINNER

- 2 fish tacos
- 1 sweet crustless quiche

DAY 13

BREAKFAST

- 2 eggs
- 2 to 3 super simple baked pancakes
- ½ of a grapefruit

LUNCH

- Thai tuna wraps
- 1 serving of salad with lemon dressing
- 2 corn tortillas
- 1 cup of grapes

SNACK

- ¼ cup of raw unsalted nuts
- 1 apple

DINNER

- 1 serving of glazed snap peas
- 1 serving of turkey salad
- 1 100% wholewheat pitta bread
- 1 serving of berry corn cobbler

DAY 14

BREAKFAST

- Coffee with up to 200gr of non-fat milk
- 1 slice of 100% wholewheat toast with 1 tablespoon of 100% raspberry jam

LUNCH

- 1 serving of curried fish cakes, topped with ½ of a sliced avocado
- ½ of a 100% wholewheat pitta bread

- 1 medium orange

SNACK
- 1 medium sliced apple
- 2 tablespoons peanut butter

DINNER
- 1 serving of spiced lamb burgers with 2 tablespoons of shredded cheddar cheese
- Small spinach salad with assorted veggies, like tomato, cucumber, carrot, sweet pepper, and 2 tablespoons of basic vinaigrette
- 1 serving of berry sundae

DAY 15

BREAKFAST
- 2 slices healthy French toast
- 200gr of non-fat milk

LUNCH
- 1 serving of crack slaw
- 2 tablespoons of baked aubergine sandwiches with 1 cup of baby carrots
- 1 medium peach

SNACK
- 1 apple
- ¼ cup of raw unsalted cashews (2 tablespoons)

DINNER
- 1 serving of fish with mushroom
- 1 medium baked sweet potato

- 1 cup of steamed spinach and 1 brie-stuffed apple

DAY 16

BREAKFAST
- 1 serving of protein bowl
- 2 slices of 100% wholewheat toast with 2 tablespoons of 100% fruit jam Green tea

LUNCH
- 1 serving of Greek salad with 1 tablespoon of lemon vinaigrette with 100gr grilled or baked
- 1 serving of beef brochettes
- 1 medium apple
- 20 almonds

SNACK
- 200gr of non-fat plain yoghurt
- 1 cup of mixed berries

DINNER
- 1 serving of Thai curried vegetables with shrimp and broccoli
- 1 cup of brown rice
- 1 banana

DAY 17

BREAKFAST
- 1 serving of green avocado smoothie
- Green tea

- ½ of bread
- 2 tablespoons of peanut butter

LUNCH

- 1 baked trout
- ½ cup of grandma's guacamole
- 1 medium orange

SNACK

- ½ cup of sliced strawberries
- ½ cup of sliced apple

DINNER

- 1 serving of lamb with prunes
- 1 serving of salad with 2 tablespoons of lemon dressing
- Vinaigrette
- ½ of a 100% wholewheat pitta bread
- 1 serving of chocolate smoothie

DAY 18

BREAKFAST

- 1 serving of melon mélange smoothie
- 2 to 3 fluffy homemade buttermilk pancakes

LUNCH

- 1 serving of lemony lentil salad with salmon
- 1 cup of grapes

SNACK

- 1 serving of dry-rubbed barbecue turkey wings
- ½ cup of baby carrots
- ½ of a sliced medium apple

DINNER

- 1 serving of jicama noodles
- 1 medium mashed sweet potato with 1 teaspoon of butter
- 1 serving of salad with 1 tablespoon of lemon dressing
- 1 cup of mixed berries

DAY 19

BREAKFAST

- 1 serving of turkey breakfast burritos
- 200gr of non-fat milk or coffee with up to 200 gr of non-fat milk
- 1 cup of mixed berries

LUNCH

- 1 serving of salad with 1 tablespoon of basic vinaigrette
- 1 medium apple

SNACK

- 1 cup of sweet popcorn balls with 1 teaspoon of butter
- 1 medium orange

DINNER

- Crab cake
- 1 serving of shrimp and broccoli
- 1 serving of chocolate dessert smoothie

DAY 20

BREAKFAST
- 2 to 3 fluffy homemade pancakes
- 200gr of non-fat milk
- ½ of a grapefruit

LUNCH
- 1 serving of salad with 1 tablespoon of basic vinaigrette
- Baked trout
- 1 cup of grapes

SNACK
- 2 sweet and nutty protein bars
- 2 tablespoons hazelnuts

DINNER
- 2 servings of chow mein
- Grilled or roasted boneless, skinless chicken breast
- 2 servings of salad with 2 tablespoons of lemon dressing

DAY 21

BREAKFAST
- 1 serving of chocolate smoothie and quick and easy apple oatmeal custard
- Coffee with up to 200gr of non-fat milk

LUNCH
- Lemon and thyme lamb chops
- Salad with 2 tablespoons of vinaigrette
- 1 medium peach

SNACK
- 1 medium apple with 2 tablespoons of peanut butter

DINNER
- 2 to 3 mushroom tacos
- 1 serving of grilled sweet potato steak fries
- ¾ cup of strawberries with homemade whipped cream

DAY 22

BREAKFAST
- 2 slices of 100% wholewheat bread
- 50gr of goat cheese

LUNCH
- 1 serving of tuna salad with 1 ½ cups of spinach
- ½ of a sliced avocado
- ½ cup of cherry tomatoes
- 1 cup of mixed berries

SNACK
- 2 crispy cauliflower filo cups

DINNER
- 1 serving of vegetable masala
- 1 cup of brown rice
- ½ cup of strawberries with 1 tablespoon of homemade whipped cream

DAY 23

BREAKFAST
- 1 tablespoon of sliced almonds and 2 to 3 simple pancakes
- Coffee or tea with 200gr of non-fat milk

LUNCH
- 1 Thai tuna wrap
- 1 medium orange

SNACK
- 2 heavenly devilled eggs
- ½ cup of grapes

DINNER
- 1 cup of white fish soup
- 1 serving of country fried steak
- 2 slices of pineapple

DAY 24

BREAKFAST
- 1 serving of tofu breakfast scramble
- ½ of a grapefruit
- Green tea

LUNCH
- Beef croquettes
- A small salad with 1 cup of mixed greens, cherry tomatoes, and sliced cucumber
- 1 medium orange

SNACK
- Orange and cinnamon biscotti
- 1 cup of carrots and sliced sweet pepper

DINNER
- 1 serving of baked sole with caramelised onion
- 6 small roasted red potatoes
- 1 small apple with 1 tablespoon of chocolate

DAY 25

BREAKFAST
- 1 egg and sausage breakfast sandwich
- 200gr of non-fat milk

LUNCH
- 1 serving of farro salad with 100gr grilled or roasted boneless, skinless chicken breast (50gr)
- 1 medium orange

SNACK
- 1 serving of shrimp spread with crackers
- 1 cup of grapes

DINNER
- 2 mushroom tacos
- 1 serving of salad with 1 tablespoon of vinaigrette

DAY 26

BREAKFAST
- 1 hard-boiled egg
- ½ of a grapefruit
- Coffee with 100gr of non-fat milk, or green tea with lemon

LUNCH
- 1 serving of baked aubergine slices with minty olive salad

SNACK
- 200gr of non-fat plain Greek yoghurt with a ½ cup of blueberries

DINNER
- 1 serving of roast beef
- 1 slice of 100% wholewheat bread
- 2 slices of fresh pineapple
- 200ml of sparkling water

DAY 27

BREAKFAST
- 1 serving of chocolate smoothie
- 1 egg and sausage breakfast sandwich

LUNCH
- ½ cup of black beans and 2 tablespoons of cheddar cheese, ½ of a sliced avocado
- Salad with 2 tablespoons of basic vinaigrette

SNACK
- 20 hazelnuts
- 200gr of non-fat plain yoghurt
- ½ cup of sliced strawberries

DINNER
- 1 serving of turkey salad
- 1 serving of grilled fish and vegetable parcels
- 1 medium baked sweet potato
- 1 serving of berry cobbler

DAY 28

BREAKFAST
- Loaded veggie eggs
- 2 tablespoons of peanut butter

LUNCH
- 1 serving of chow mein
- 200 gr of non-fat milk
- 1 medium orange

SNACK
- 1 cup of cherries
- 20 almonds

DINNER
- 1 serving of pasta salad
- 1 serving of homemade burger
- 1 cup of frozen grapes

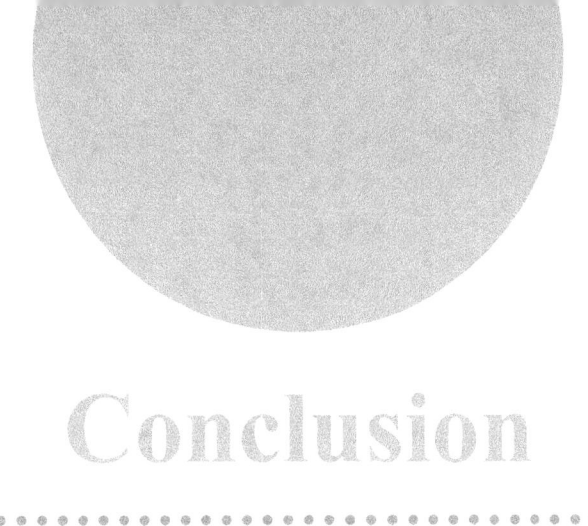

Conclusion

A person may prevent or reduce some health problems linked with CKD by eating the right meals and avoiding foods high in salt, potassium, and phosphorus. The renal diet is the greatest option since it maintains kidney function while delaying the progression of total kidney failure. It stresses the need to eat high-quality protein and limit liquid consumption. The nutritious nature of keto acid supplements and the renal diet can have a preventive role for cardiovascular diseases in patients with chronic renal disease. It impacts traditional and non-traditional cardiovascular risks when combined with a diet that restricts phosphorus, protein, and sodium. Decreasing salt, potassium, and phosphorus consumption may help control blood pressure, which is important for lowering serum cholesterol and improving plasma lipid profiles. Low protein and phosphorus consumption is critical for preventing and treating proteinuria, hypophosphatemia and secondary hyperparathyroidism. These are the primary causes of vascular calcification, heart diseases, and uremic mortality.

Leaving aside the previously contested effect on renal disease progression, proper nutritional treatment or a kidney-friendly diet, such as the renal diet, may help decrease the risk of cardiovascular disease in people with renal disease early on. As stated at the beginning of this book, patients with reduced renal function should choose foods and diet plans cautiously.

Finally, the healthiest diet for renal diseases and other health problems is the one that a person can establish and sustain a healthy lifestyle with. Thus, the renal diet is a powerful and effective method for dealing with critical renal diseases like CKD while remaining healthy and enjoying your favourite foods.

The kidney-friendly foods mentioned in this book are great options for those on a renal diet. Always consult with your healthcare professional about your dietary choices before making any changes. This is to guarantee that you implement the optimal diet for your specific requirements. Dietary limitations differ based on the type and severity of kidney disease and the medical procedures used, such as the medicines used or dialysis. While adhering to a renal diet may seem restrictive at points, many tasty items can be included in a healthy, nutritious, well-balanced diet plan that supports your kidneys.

Recipes Index

- Almond Meringue Cookies — 32
- Apple and Blueberry Crisp — 31
- Baked Lamb Chops — 78
- Baked sole with caramelized onion — 60
- Baked Sweet Potato Chips — 43
- Beans and Cucumber Salad — 58
- Beef brochettes — 72
- Beef pot roast — 74
- Blueberry Corn Cobbler — 28
- Broccoli and Apple Salad — 47
- Cheese and Asparagus Crepe Rolls with Parsley — 26
- Chicken and Mandarin Salad — 46
- chickpea and avocado salads — 41
- Chinese beef wraps — 69
- Cilantro Chili Burgers — 54
- Country fried steak — 73
- Cranberry Dip with Fresh Fruit — 36
- Cranberry Lemon Parfait — 34
- Egg and Sausage Breakfast Sandwich — 25
- Fish taco — 66
- Fluffy Homemade Buttermilk Pancakes — 20
- Fresh Berry Fruit Salad with Yogurt Cream — 30
- Glazed Snap Peas — 52
- Greek Yogurt Berry Parfait — 42
- Grilled fish and vegetable packets — 62
- Grilled Lamb Chops with Pineapple — 79
- Grilled skirt steak — 70
- Homemade burgers — 75
- Homemade Herbed Biscuits — 40
- Jicama Noodles — 55
- Lemon butter salmon — 63
- Loaded Veggie Eggs — 23
- Minty Olives Salad — 57
- Mushroom Tacos — 56
- Oatmeal with Honey and Fruit — 22
- Orange and Cinnamon Biscotti — 39
- Pasta Salad — 48
- Peppercorn Pork Chops — 76
- Pork Chops with Apples, Onions — 77
- Pork loins with leeks — 68
- Proteins Booster Blueberry Muffins — 29
- Raspberry Cheesecake Mousse — 33
- Roast beef — 71
- Roasted Red Pepper Hummus with Veggie Sticks — 49
- Salad with Lemon Dressing — 45
- Shrimp & broccoli — 64
- Shrimp in garlic sauce — 65
- Shrimp Spread with Crackers — 37
- Soft Ginger Cookies — 38
- Stuffed Breakfast Biscuits — 21
- Super Simple Baked Pancake — 24
- Thai tuna wraps — 61
- Turkey Salad — 50
- Vegetable Masala — 53

www.ingramcontent.com/pod-product-compliance
Lightning Source LLC
Chambersburg PA
CBHW081549240526
45470CB00024B/2721